PHARMACOPŒA GERMANICA.

THE

GERMAN PHARMACOPŒIA.

TRANSLATED BY

C. L. LOCHMAN.

WITH

AN APPENDIX

EXPLANATORY OF THE FRENCH METRICAL SYSTEM, AND TABLES OF WEIGHTS AND MEASURES, ETC.

PHILADELPHIA:
DAVID D. ELDER & CO.,
430 Market Street.
1873.

Entered, according to Act of Congress, in the year 1873, by

C. L. LOCHMAN,

in the Office of the Librarian of Congress, at Washington, D. C.

PHILADELPHIA
PRINTED BY SHERMAN & CO.

INTRODUCTION

BY THE TRANSLATOR.

The fact that hitherto no English translation has existed of any of the Pharmacopœias of the German States, and that they were almost sealed books to many American pharmacists, has induced the translator to prepare one of the "*Pharmacopœa Germanica*," or German Pharmacopœia, which has recently taken the place of the various Pharmacopœias of the German States, and is now the only legally recognized Pharmacopœia for the whole German empire.

The Pharmacopœia was compiled, after the establishment of the Empire, by gentlemen of acknowledged ability in the various departments of science, in Germany.

It will be appreciated for its concise, accurate, and scientific descriptions of *Materia Medica* and preparations; giving briefly the characteristic marks by which the purity and identity of a drug may be readily ascertained.

In view of the already large, and rapidly increasing German population, including many physicians, the work, it is hoped, will be acceptable to many pharmacists, who are frequently called upon for medicines by the German names, or by the Latin terms, in use in Germany.

In the English translation of officinal terms, especially of chemistry, the nomenclature adopted in the late United States Pharmacopœia (Revision of 1870), has been followed, as far as practicable. It must be remembered, however, that many preparations, though bearing similar names to those of the

United States Pharmacopœia, are not of equal strength, and many liquids vary in specific gravity, and that the articles named, have reference to each other only in this Pharmacopœia, and do not refer to any other.

The metrical system of weights and measures is established by law in the German empire; but in the formulas of this work, the quantity of every article is given in *parts* by *weight*, and in no case by *measure of capacity*. The temperatures are expressed in degrees of the centigrade (Celsius') thermometer. The specific gravity of liquids are taken at 15° of that scale.

The manner of preserving articles "*cautiously*" or "*very cautiously*," has reference to the separation and seclusion of medicines, according to the instructions given at the heads of Tables B and C.

The Latin and German names of the various medicines contained in the Pharmacopœia, at the head of each article, with their synonyms, have been strictly adhered to, and the English terms and synonyms are designated by being inclosed in brackets [—].

To the Latin and German indexes, a full English index has been added, as well as one of systematic names of the plants and animals which furnish the articles of the materia medica. The latter index is not found in the original work, but it was considered of sufficient importance to be inserted in the translation.

An Appendix, explanatory of the centigrade and Fahrenheit's thermometers, and of the French metrical system of weights and measures, has also been added, together with comparative tables of weights and measures, and tables of weights and measures of the United States and British Pharmacopœias.

The preface to the original work will explain the scope of the Pharmacopœia, the various tables admitted, and under what auspices it has been prepared.

The translator hopes that the spirit of the age, which has brought about the formation of common Pharmacopœias for

NOTICE OF THE PUBLICATION

OF THE

PHARMACOPŒA GERMANICA,

OF JUNE 1, 1872.

By virtue of a resolution of the Federal Council, (Bundesrathe) passed at its session on May 22d, of this year (1872), it is hereby made public, that the Book of Medicines, which, under the title of "*Pharmacopœa Germanica*," has been adopted by a committee, appointed by the Federal Council, and which has been published at the Royal Prussian Printing-Office, of R. von Decker, at Berlin, shall take the place of the different Pharmacopœias in use in the several States of the Confederacy, from the first of November of this year.

For the Chancellor of the Empire,

Signed by

DELBRÜCK.

BERLIN, June 1, 1872.

whole empires, such as the British and the German, may, at no distant day, induce the enlightened nations of the earth to adopt a UNIVERSAL PHARMACOPŒIA upon a basis broad enough to suit all nationalities, and to accept a uniform system of weights and measures, so as to bring about unity and harmony of the present incongruous systems of weights and measures, terminology, and medicines of various strength which bear similar names, all of which are liable to lead to serious errors.

Finally, the translator would avail himself of the present opportunity of expressing his obligations to Mr. H. M. Wilder, of Philadelphia, who kindly read over the whole manuscript, and compared it critically with the original Latin text; and for the warm interest he has taken in the progress of the work, and especially for the labor bestowed on the revision of the proof-sheets.

CARLISLE, PA., November, 1873.

PREFACE.

THE want of a Pharmacopœia, that should be recognized as authority throughout Germany, having been felt for a long time, at the request of many persons, the Pharmaceutical Societies, one of which exists in North Germany and the other in South Germany, prepared a National Pharmacopœia, which appeared in an improved form in the year 1867, under the title of "*Pharmacopœa Germaniæ;*" and it was presented to the Cabinets of the various States of Germany for inspection, and, should it appear suitable, for formal adoption.

The authorities of Mecklenburg-Schwerin, having called the attention of the Federal Council, after the formation of the North German Confederacy, to the want of a common Pharmacopœia, the matter was considered, and on the 19th of December, 1868, it was resolved that a committee of physicians and pharmacists should be chosen, whose duty it should be to compile such a Pharmacopœia. The committee, having assembled on the 28th of May, 1869, concluded that not only the Prussian Pharmacopœia but the Pharmacopœia of Germany (*Pharmacopœa Germaniæ*), should be laid under contribution; and it was resolved, in regard to the medicines to be introduced into the Pharmacopœia, to get the opinions of all the physicians and pharmacists throughout the North German Confederacy, who enjoy a reputation and are of acknowledged authority. The enterprise was interrupted by the operations of the war, but after the establishment of the German Empire it was taken up again.

In pursuance of a decree, passed by the Federal Council, on the 29th of April, 1871, a committee was chosen anew, to prepare a Pharmacopœia. The committee was also joined by scientists from South Germany, to whom was committed the same charge.

The work was commenced in September, 1871, with the assistance of gentlemen from all parts of Germany, who enjoyed the highest reputation in the different departments of science. The committee brought their labors to a close in December of the same year.

It is apparent that this Pharmacopœia, in the full sense of the word, is not a new one; nor was it the intention of the committee to produce such a one. The main object was to collect the formulas of the different Pharmacopœias in a critical manner, and, as it were, to remodel the Prussian Pharmacopœia, as well as the Pharmacopœia of Germany ("*Pharmacopœa Germaniæ*"), without leaving unnoticed the recognized Pharmacopœias of South Germany.

The new Pharmacopœia became larger by the introduction and description of many simple articles and preparations, which have been recognized of late as excellent remedial agents. It was concluded to retain the Latin language, partly because it is everywhere understood, and partly because physicians prefer to write their prescriptions in that language.

As it was necessary to decide what medicines should be introduced into the Pharmacopœia, in general, proper attention was paid to all suggestions and wishes that came under notice from the different parts of Germany.

The contents of our Pharmacopœia will, no doubt, at the present time, offer all that is considered necessary to the pharmacists of Germany. But as the articles are numerous and varied, it was not considered proper to compel the pharmacists to keep on hand all the simple articles or preparations adopted by the Pharmacopœia. It cannot, therefore, be definitely stated which articles should be kept by the pharmacists in general: that matter must be left to be determined by the various States, according to the wants of the different localities.

With regard to the form and arrangement of this Pharmacopœia, the compilers have followed former works of this kind;

the alphabetical order has been retained, and, for the most part, the customary officinal names of the remedies prepared from plants. On the contrary, as regards either simple articles or chemical preparations, it was considered preferable to retain the names which had been in common use for a long time by physicians and pharmacists, and which are also used in medical and pharmacological works.

After the proper title at the head of each article, beside the German names, there are given also such synonyms as were considered of importance.

Where it treats of simple articles, whether derived from vegetables or animals, the descriptions must necessarily be short, but they are given with the utmost accuracy, as to the characteristic marks, and stating also when the indigenous plants, necessary to the pharmacist, should be collected.

As most of the chemical preparations are made in a better and more scientific manner in the chemical establishments, it was left to the pharmacist to draw his chemicals from those sources or from dealers. Only certain directions are given in our Pharmacopœia for the preparation of such chemicals as differ in composition, when prepared by different formulas.

Since the pharmacists are held responsible for the quality and purity of all articles they keep on hand, brief methods are given by which each chemical is to be tested, to establish fully its purity and identity.

For this purpose are added to the Pharmacopœia the names of reagents, and of what concentration they should be, so that the investigation may be properly carried out.

Finally, at the end of the work the following tables will be found:

1. Table A, consisting of remedies which are of considerable therapeutic power and activity, giving the maximum doses, both in the largest single dose, and the largest quantity that may be administered during a period of twenty-four hours.

2. In the tables B and C are enumerated the remedies which are to be cautiously preserved, and kept separate from the

others, namely: such as are usually termed poisons, and such as are possessed of very great therapeutic power and activity.

3. The table following gives the specific gravities of the liquid remedies. The temperature of 15° of Celsius' (centigrade) scale has been established as the point at which the specific gravity is to be taken, to which point all liquids to be examined, at any time of the year, can be readily brought.

4. The specific gravities of alcohol, of different strengths, are noted, and the degrees are given, which a correct areometer (hydrometer) must indicate.

The table printed at the beginning of the work, gives the atomic weights of the different elements which are found in the chemical formulas in the Pharmacopœia.

A table of weights, which must be used in the shops, was considered superfluous, as such weights are established by law throughout the German Empire.

Finally, in order to find readily each separate article, treated of in this work, two very accurate indexes are attached, one of which gives the German names, and the other the Latin terms of the remedies.

Berlin, May, 1872.

SYMBOLS AND ATOMIC WEIGHTS OF THE ELEMENTS

AS USED IN THIS PHARMACOPŒIA.

Elements.	Symbols.	Atomic Weight.
Aluminum,	Al	27.4
Antimony (Stibium),	Sb	122.0
Arsenicum,	As	75.0
Barium,	Ba	137.0
Bismuth,	Bi	210.0
Bromine,	Br	80.0
Calcium,	Ca	40.0
Carbon,	C	12.0
Chlorine,	Cl	35.5
Chromium,	Cr	52.0
Copper,	Cu	63.5
Gold,	Au	197.0
Hydrogen,	H	1.0
Iodine,	I	127.0
Iron,	Fe	56.0
Lead,	Pb	207.0
Lithium,	Li	7.0
Magnesium,	Mg	24.0
Manganese,	Mn	55.0
Mercury,	Hg	200.0
Nitrogen,	N	14.0
Oxygen,	O	16.0
Phosphorus,	P	31.0
Potassium (Kalium),	K	39.0
Silver,	Ag	108.0
Sodium (Natrium),	Na	23.0
Sulphur,	S	32.0
Tin,	Sn	118.0
Zinc,	Zn	65.0

The quantity of liquids, indicated by "parts," is always to be determined by weight, and never by measure.

THE

GERMAN PHARMACOPŒIA.

Acetum.

[VINEGAR]. Essig.

Acetum crudum. Acetum Vini.

A transparent, colorless or slightly yellowish liquid, of a purely sour taste and odor. *Twenty parts* of vinegar should contain sufficient [acetic] acid to saturate *one part* of anhydrous carbonate of sodium.

It should contain no free sulphuric or other foreign acids.

Acetum aromaticum.

[AROMATIC VINEGAR]. Aromatischer Essig.

Take of	Oil of Rosemary, ...	1
	Oil of Juniper, ...	1
	Oil of Lemon, each, *one part*, ...	1
	Oil of Thyme *two parts*, ...	2
	Oil of Cloves *five parts*, ...	5
	Tincture of Cinnamon *one hundred parts*, .	100
	Aromatic Tincture *fifty parts*, ...	50
	Diluted Acetic Acid *two hundred parts*, . .	200
	Distilled Water *one thousand parts*. . . .	1000

Mix, and keep for three days in a cool place, then filter.

It should be a clear, brownish-red liquid, of an agreeably sour and aromatic odor.

Acetum Colchici.

[Vinegar of Colchicum]. Zeitlosenessig.

Take of Colchicum Seed, bruised,	1
Alcohol, each, *one part*,	1
Pure Vinegar *nine parts*.	9

Digest for eight days, then express and filter.
Vinegar of colchicum is a clear, yellowish liquid.
It should be *cautiously* preserved.

Acetum Digitalis.

[Vinegar of Digitalis]. Fingerhutessig.

Take of Digitalis Leaves, cut,	1
Alcohol, each, *one part*,	1
Pure Vinegar *nine parts*.	9

Macerate for eight days, express and filter.
Vinegar of digitalis is a clear, reddish liquid.
It should be *cautiously* preserved.

Acetum purum.

[Pure Vinegar]. Reiner Essig.

Acetum destillatum.

Take of Diluted Acetic Acid *one part*,	1
Distilled Water *four parts*.	4

Mix them.

A transparent, colorless liquid, of a purely sour taste and smell. It should contain *six per cent.* of acetic acid, so that *twenty parts* are sufficient to saturate *one part* of anhydrous carbonate of sodium.

Acetum pyrolignosum crudum.

[Crude Wood Vinegar]. Roher Holzessig.

A brownish, or brown liquid, containing acetic acid, and having an empyreumatic odor. *Twenty parts* should be sufficient to saturate *one part* of anhydrous carbonate of sodium.

Acetum pyrolignosum rectificatum.

[RECTIFIED WOOD VINEGAR]. Rectificirter Holzessig.

From *ten parts* of Crude Wood Vinegar, introduced into a glass retort, *eight parts* are drawn off by distillation.

It forms a clear, colorless, or a yellowish or slightly brownish liquid, of an empyreumatic odor, and a smoky, acid taste.

It should be preserved in well-stopped bottles.

Acetum Rubi Idæi.

[VINEGAR OF RASPBERRY]. Himbeeressig.

Take of Syrup of Raspberry *one part*, ...	1
Pure Vinegar *two parts*.	2

Mix them.

It is prepared only when wanted for dispensing.

Acetum Scillæ.

[VINEGAR OF SQUILL]. Meerzwiebelessig.

Acetum Scilliticum.

Take of Squill, dry and cut in small pieces, ...	1
Alcohol, each, *one part*, ...	1
Pure Vinegar *nine parts*.	9

Macerate for three days, shaking frequently, then express and filter.

It forms a clear, yellowish liquid.

It should be preserved in well-stopped bottles.

Acidum aceticum.

[GLACIAL ACETIC ACID]. Essigsäure.

Acidum aceticum concentratum. Acetum glaciale.

A colorless, transparent liquid, of a pungent, acid smell, which above 0° C.* becomes a crystalline mass, but regains its fluidity at a temperature of 16° C.; at 118° C. it boils and volatilizes entirely. *Ten parts* should dissolve *one part* of oil of lemon. By the addition of a few drops of solution of permanganate of potassium, a permanent red color is produced. Acetic acid, diluted with twenty parts of water, should not

---

* The translator has added the letter C. throughout the work, to the number of degrees, to indicate the Centigrade Scale.

become turbid on the addition of chloride of barium, nitrate of silver, or hydrosulphuric acid.*

It should be preserved in glass-stoppered bottles.

Acidum aceticum aromaticum.

[AROMATIC ACETIC ACID]. Gewürzhafte Essigsäure.

Take of Oil of Cloves *nine parts*,	9
Oil of Lavender,	6
Oil of Lemon, each, *six parts*,	6
Oil of Bergamot,	3
Oil of Thyme, each, *three parts*,	3
Oil of Cinnamon *one part*.	1
Dissolve, by agitation, in	
Acetic Acid *twenty-five parts*.	25

It forms a clear, brownish-yellow liquid.

Acidum aceticum dilutum.

[DILUTED ACETIC ACID]. Verdünnte Essigsäure.

Acetum concentratum.

A colorless, transparent liquid, of a very sour taste, having a pungent acid odor, free from empyreuma. The specific gravity is 1.040. *One thousand parts* are sufficient to saturate *two hundred and sixty-five* (265) *parts* of anhydrous carbonate of sodium, corresponding to thirty per cent. of acetic acid.

It behaves, in the presence of reagents, like acetic acid.

Acidum arsenicosum.

[ARSENIOUS ACID]. Arsenige Säure.

[***White Arsenic***]. ***Weisser Arsenik.*** ***Arsenicum album.***

For medical purposes, only that which consists of whitish, more or less opaque pieces, and not the powder, should be employed.

By a strong heat it is entirely volatilized, in the form of white fumes; it dissolves slowly in water, without a residue.

It should be preserved *very cautiously*.

---

* For the sake of brevity, the term "hydrosulphuric acid" is employed, in the translation, for "aqueous solution of hydrosulphuric acid," or "sulphuretted hydrogen water"—"aqua hydrosulphurata" (Schwefelwasserstoffwasser, *Germ.*), in the original.

Acidum benzoicum.

[SUBLIMED BENZOIC ACID]. Sublimirte Benzoesäure.

Acidum benzoicum sublimatum. Flores Benzoes.

It is prepared by sublimation from Benzoin.

It consists of white crystals, which change by age to a yellowish color; they are of a silky lustre, having the odor of benzoin; readily soluble in two hundred parts of cold, and twenty-five parts of boiling water; also, in alcohol, ether, oil of turpentine, and in water of ammonia. When heated, they first melt and are afterwards wholly volatilized.

A hot aqueous solution of the crystals must not evolve the odor of bitter almonds, when heated with permanganate of potassium.

It should be preserved in well-closed vessels.

Acidum boricum.

[BORACIC ACID]. Borsäure.

Acidum boracicum. Sal sedativum Hombergii.

In white, pearly, crystalline scales, which have scarcely an acid taste; when heated they first melt with disengagement of watery vapor, and then fuse into a mass, which, on cooling, hardens into a transparent glass.

It is soluble in twenty-six parts of cold, and three parts of boiling water, and also in alcohol. An aqueous solution should not become turbid on the addition of nitrate of silver, or chloride of barium; nor should it assume a red color with sulphocyanide of potassium.

Acidum carbolicum crudum.

[CRUDE CARBOLIC ACID]. Rohe Carbolsäure.

[***Impure Carbolic Acid***].

A reddish-brown, more or less transparent liquid, of a strongly empyreumatic smell; slightly soluble in water, more freely in alcohol, and almost entirely so in a hot solution of caustic soda. It should contain, at least, *fifty per cent.* of pure carbolic acid.

Acidum carbolicum crystallisatum.

[CRYSTALLIZED CARBOLIC ACID. PURE CARBOLIC ACID].
Carbolsäure.

[Phenic Acid]. Phenol. Acidum phenylicum. Phenylsäure.

A crystalline, neutral, colorless or slightly reddish mass; consisting of long-pointed crystals, of a peculiar odor and very acrid taste. When exposed to fire it burns with a white flame; melts between 25° and 30° C. (the pure and anhydrous at 42°), and boils at about 180° C. It is slightly soluble in cold water, and mixes in all proportions with ether, chloroform, bisulphide of carbon and glycerin. Shaken with chloroform or bisulphide of carbon, on account of the presence of a small quantity of water, it becomes somewhat cloudy. It has the specific gravity of about 1.060, when fused.

When shaken with no less than fifty parts, or at most sixty parts of cold water, or with a small quantity of solution of caustic soda, it yields a clear solution. The aqueous solution is colored violet, when mixed with a few drops of solution of sesquichloride of iron, which color lasts for some time.

It should be *cautiously* preserved.

Acidum chloro-nitrosum.

[NITRO-MURIATIC ACID]. Königswasser.

Aqua regia.

Take of Pure Hydrochloric Acid *three parts*, . . . 3
Pure nitric Acid *one part*. 1

Mix them.

It is only prepared when wanted for dispensing.

Acidum chromicum.

[CHROMIC ACID]. Chromsäure.

In columnar or needle-form, frequently pointed crystals of a scarlet-red color; inodorous; deliquescent in the air, and freely soluble in water and alcohol. When heated, they become black, then melt and yield oxygen.

An aqueous solution, when boiled for some time with hydrochloric acid and a little alcohol; must not turn very turbid on the addition of chloride of barium.

It should be *cautiously* preserved.

Acidum citricum.

[CITRIC ACID]. Citronensäure.

In colorless, translucent, rhombic-prismatic crystals; permanent in the air, freely soluble in water, and alcohol, but insoluble in ether; they effloresce at a moderate heat, melt at a higher temperature, and are charred at a red heat. A solution, mixed with an excess of lime water, and heated, yields a white precipitate, which disappears again on cooling.

An aqueous solution should not be rendered turbid by hydrosulphuric acid, nitrate of barium, acetate of potassium, oxalate of ammonium, or sulphate of calcium.

Acidum hydrochloricum.

[PURE HYDROCHLORIC ACID]. Reine Salzsäure.

[*Pure Muriatic Acid*]. *Acidum hydrochloratum.* *Acidum muriaticum.*

A colorless, transparent liquid, entirely volatilized by heat, having the specific gravity of 1.124, and containing *twenty-five* per cent. of anhydrous hydrochloric acid. When diluted with five parts of distilled water, no change should be produced by hydrosulphuric acid, nor should it become turbid with chloride of barium, turn red with sulphocyanide of potassium, or blue by a mixture of starch paste and iodide of potassium.

To test it for sulphurous or arsenious acid:—put a few small pieces of pure zinc into a rather long test-tube, and introduce the hydrochloric acid, diluted with two parts of water, which should fill about one-tenth part of the tube; into the upper portion of the tube is placed a pellet of cotton-wool, saturated with a solution of acetate of lead, and the mouth of the vessel is covered with a piece of white bibulous paper, moistened with a solution of nitrate of silver. After an active evolution of gas, for half an hour, in the absence of sulphurous or arsenious acid, neither the cotton nor the paper is blackened.

It should be *cautiously* preserved in glass-stoppered bottles.

Acidum hydrochloricum crudum.

[CRUDE HYDROCHLORIC ACID]. Rohe Salzsäure.

Acidum hydrochloratum crudum.

[***Crude Muriatic Acid***]. ***Acidum muriaticum crudum.*** ***Spiritus salis.***

A transparent, yellowish, fuming liquid, of from 1.160 to 1.170 specific gravity, corresponding to thirty and thirty-three per cent. of anhydrous hydrochloric acid. It contains traces of sulphuric and sulphurous acids, alumina and iron.

An acid, contaminated with arsenious acid, must be rejected. It is tested as follows:—about ten grammes of the acid, after adding one gramme of protochloride of tin, is either heated or set aside for half an hour. The hydrochloric acid contaminated with arsenious acid, will then, on account of liberated metallic arsenic, become turbid and brown.

It should be *cautiously* preserved.

Acidum hydrochloricum dilutum.

[DILUTED HYDROCHLORIC ACID]. Verdünnte Salzsäure.

[***Diluted Muriatic Acid***].

Take of Pure Hydrochloric Acid,
Distilled Water, each, *equal parts.*

Mix them.

It forms a colorless, transparent liquid, having the specific gravity 1.060.

It should be preserved in glass-stoppered bottles.

Acidum lacticum.

[LACTIC ACID]. Milchsäure.

A clear, colorless, or yellowish, syrupy, inodorous liquid, of a sour taste, having the specific gravity 1.24. It is charred by a strong heat, burns with a bright flame, and is volatilized without residue. It is soluble in water, alcohol, and in ether. When mixed with solution of permanganate of potassium, and heated, it emits the odor of aldehyd. If diluted with water, it must not become turbid by hydrosulphuric acid, chloride of barium, nitrate of silver, or oxalate of ammonium. On being heated it gives off no odor of acetic or butyric acid.

Acidum nitricum.

[PURE NITRIC ACID]. Reine Salpetersäure.

A colorless transparent liquid, wholly volatilized by heat; having the specific gravity 1.185, corresponding to *thirty per cent.* of nitric acid (NHO_3).

The acid, diluted with an equal quantity of distilled water, must not immediately assume a violet-red color on the addition of a few drops of chloroform, nor after the addition of hydrosulphuric acid. Diluted with five parts of distilled water, it must not become turbid with nitrate of barium or nitrate of silver, nor be colored red by sulphocyanide of potassium.

It should be *cautiously* preserved in glass-stoppered bottles.

Acidum nitricum crudum.

[AQUA FORTIS]. Scheidewasser.

It is colorless or yellowish, and is volatilized by heat without a residue; specific gravity of from 1.323 to 1.331, corresponding to fifty and fifty-two per cent. of nitric acid (NHO_3).

It should be *cautiously* preserved.

Acidum nitricum dilutum.

[DILUTED NITRIC ACID]. Verdünnte Salpetersäure.

Take of Pure Nitric Acid,
Distilled Water, each, *equal parts.*

Mix them.

A colorless, transparent liquid; specific gravity of from 1.086 to 1.089.

It should be preserved in glass-stoppered bottles.

Acidum nitricum fumans.

[FUMING NITRIC ACID]. Rauchende Salpetersäure.

Acidum nitroso—nitricum. Spiritus nitri fumans.

A transparent, brownish-red liquid, emitting red suffocating fumes; specific gravity of from 1.520 to 1.525.

If largely diluted with water, it must become but slightly turbid with nitrate of silver or nitrate of barium.

It should be *cautiously* preserved in glass-stoppered bottles.

Acidum phosphoricum.

[PHOSPHORIC ACID]. Phosphorsäure.

A colorless, transparent, and inodorous liquid, of a sour taste, having the specific gravity of 1.120, which corresponds to twenty per cent. of phosphoric acid (PH_3O_4).

When nearly saturated with carbonate of sodium, it yields, on the addition of nitrate of silver, a light-yellow precipitate, which is completely soluble in nitric acid, and in water of ammonia. It must not become turbid when saturated with hydrosulphuric acid gas, and kept for a considerable time in a closed vessel. If it be colored by the addition of a few drops of solution of permanganate of potassium, or solution of indigo, and heated, it must in neither case become discolored. The diluted acid should not be rendered very turbid by nitrate of barium.

The acid, evaporated to one-fifth of its weight, may be used in place of *dry* or *glacial* phosphoric acid (*Acidum phosphoricum siccum s. glaciale*), when the latter is prescribed in a pill mass.

Acidum succinicum.

[SUCCINIC ACID]. Bernsteinsäure.

Sal succini volatile.

It occurs in crusts of cohering, yellowish crystals, having the odor of oil of amber. When exposed to heat, it is entirely volatilized, giving out fumes that provoke coughing. It is soluble in twenty-eight parts of cold water, 2.2 of boiling water, freely in alcohol, and very slightly in ether, but insoluble in oil of turpentine.

A concentrated aqueous solution produces with solution of acetate of potassium no crystalline precipitate. It is not rendered turbid by chloride of barium, or chloride of calcium, nor altered by hydrosulphuric acid. When colored with a few drops of indigo solution, it is not discolored by the addition of sulphuric acid when heated. The acid rubbed with caustic lime must not yield an ammoniacal odor.

Acidum sulfuricum.

[PURE SULPHURIC ACID]. Reine Schwefelsäure.

Acidum sulfuricum rectificatum.

A colorless, inodorous liquid, of an oily consistence, entirely volatilized by heat, having the specific gravity 1.840, which corresponds to 98.5 per cent. of sulphuric acid (SH_2O_4).

When mixed with three times its volume of alcohol, it yields no precipitate; diluted with water, it is not affected by hydrosulphuric acid; it does not change the color of indigo solution, nor discolor a solution of permanganate of potassium when heated. It should not contain arsenious acid, which is ascertained by the method used in testing pure hydrochloric acid, excepting that the sulphuric acid be previously diluted with five or six parts of water.

It should be *cautiously* preserved in glass-stoppered bottles.

Acidum sulfuricum crudum.

[CRUDE SULPHURIC ACID]. Rohe Schwefelsäure.

Englische Schwefelsäure.

A transparent, generally colorless liquid, of an oily consistence; specific gravity of from 1.830 to 1.833, corresponding to 91.8 and 93.1 per cent. of sulphuric acid (SH_2O_4). Diluted with five parts of water and filtered, then saturated with hydrosulphuric acid gas, it should not yield, in a warm place, a yellow precipitate, which is easily soluble in a solution of carbonate of ammonium.

It should be *cautiously* preserved in glass-stoppered bottles.

Acidum sulfuricum dilutum.

[DILUTED SULPHURIC ACID]. Verdünnte Schwefelsäure.

Take of Pure Sulphuric Acid *one part*, ... 1
Distilled water *five parts*. 5

The acid is dropped cautiously and gradually into the water while it is stirred with a glass rod. The specific gravity ranges from 1.113 to 1.117.

Acidum sulfuricum fumans.

[FUMING SULPHURIC ACID]. Rauchende Schwefelsäure.

[Nordhausen Oil of Vitriol]. Nordhäuser Vitriolöl.

A brownish, oily liquid, emitting white suffocating fumes; specific gravity of from 1.860 to 1.900.

It should be tested like crude sulphuric acid.

Preserve it *cautiously* in well-closed, glass-stoppered bottles.

Acidum tannicum.

[TANNIC ACID]. Gerbsäure.

Tannin. Acidum gallo-tannicum.

A yellowish-white powder, burns when ignited, leaving no residue; freely soluble in water, less so in alcohol. It has a slight acid reaction.

The aqueous solution is entirely clear or nearly so, and on being first treated with alcohol and then with ether, it does not become turbid.

When the acid is shaken with ether, to which a small quantity of water has been added, a somewhat dense liquid is formed, which subsides in the ether.

Acidum tartaricum.

[TARTARIC ACID]. Weinsteinsäure.

Sal essentiale tartari.

In columnar, monoclinic, colorless, and inodorous crystals, frequently concreting together in crusts; they are permanent in the air, charred by heat, and burn without a residue; soluble in an equal weight of cold water, much more readily in boiling water, and in three parts of alcohol.

The acid, dissolved in double its weight of water should not become turbid by hydrosulphuric acid, nitrate of barium or oxalate of ammonium.

Acidum valerianicum.

[VALERIANIC ACID]. Baldriansäure.

A colorless, transparent liquid, of a peculiar odor, having a specific gravity of from 0.940 to 0.950 (responding to $C_5H_{10}O_2+H_2O$); soluble in all proportions of ether, alcohol, and water of ammonia.

Twenty-five parts of water scarcely dissolve one part of valerianic acid, which solution should redden blue test-paper, but should not be rendered turbid by chloride of barium or nitrate of silver.

The acid, neutralized by water of ammonia, which has been diluted with an equal volume of distilled water, yields a reddish-brown, resinous precipitate, on the addition of a few drops of solution of sesquichloride of iron, but the supernatant liquid should not assume a red color.

Preserve it in glass-stoppered bottles.

Aconitinum.

[ACONITIA OR ACONITIN]. Akonitin.

A white or yellowish-white, inodorous powder, having a bitter, followed by a sharp, taste, producing an acrid sensation in the throat. It has an alkaline reaction and is very sparingly soluble in cold water; more readily in water acidulated with hydrochloric acid. It is soluble, also, in alcohol, ether, and chloroform. It softens in hot water and runs together into a resin-like mass, which afterwards dissolves, slowly, in fifty parts of boiling water. It dissolves in sulphuric acid, with a yellowish-red color, which, after twenty-four hours, is changed to a brownish-red. When heated in a water-bath with phosphoric acid, it assumes a violet color.

It should be preserved with *great caution.*

Adeps suillus.

[LARD. HOG'S LARD]. Schweineschmalz.

Axungia porci vel porcina.

Sus scrofa *Linn.*

It should be very white, nearly inodorous, and without a rancid taste. It is prepared by rendering the fat attached to the mesentery and kidneys.

Ærugo.

[VERDIGRIS]. Grünspan.

Spangrün. Viride Æris. Cuprum subaceticum.

In the form of solid cakes or balls, of a green or bluish-green color. It is pulverized with difficulty.

Only partially soluble in water. Soluble in dilute sulphuric acid, acetic acid, and in water of ammonia; leaving only a very small quantity of impurities behind.

It should be *cautiously* preserved.

Æther.

[ETHER]. Schwefeläther.

[Sulphuric Ether]. Æther sulfuricus. Naphtha vitrioli.

A colorless, transparent liquid, which is free from acids, and is wholly volatilized in the air, so that a saturated linen cloth should be left without odor after spontaneous evaporation of the ether. The specific gravity must not exceed 0.728.

It should be preserved in rather small, well-stopped bottles, in a cool place.

Æther aceticus.

[ACETIC ETHER]. Essigäther.

Naphtha aceti.

A colorless liquid, free from acids, having the specific gravity of from 0.900 to 0.904.

When shaken with an equal volume of water, the bulk of water must not increase over one-tenth.

It should be preserved in well-closed bottles, in a cool place.

Æther petrolei.

[PETROLEUM NAPHTHA]. Petroleumäther.

A liquid procured by distillation from American petroleum.

It is transparent, colorless, and very inflammable, possessing but a slight petroleum odor. When poured drop by drop into the palm of the hand it evaporates rapidly, leaving no odor. It is not miscible with water, but swims on its surface. Its specific gravity ranges from 0.670 to 0.675 and it boils at a temperature of from 50° to 60° C. When boiled for a few minutes with a fourth of its volume of spirit of ammonia and a small quantity of nitrate of silver, the ammoniacal liquid must not turn brown.

It should be preserved in well-closed vessels, in a cool place.

Æthylenum chloratum.

[Bichloride of Ethylene]. Aethylenchlorid. Elaylchlorid.

[Dutch Liquid]. Elaylum chloratum. Liquor Hollandicus.

A clear liquid, of the odor of chloroform, having the specific gravity 1.270; boils at a temperature of 85° C.; scarcely soluble in water; freely soluble in alcohol, and in ether.

Distilled water, shaken with it, must not alter blue test-paper, nor become turbid with nitrate of silver.

It should be preserved in well-closed bottles.

Aloe.

[Aloes]. Aloe.

[Cape or Shining Aloes]. Aloe capensis vel lucida.

Aloe spicata *Thunberg* and of other species of Aloe.

In opaque, dark-brown masses, with a greenish tint, the edges viewed by transmitted light are of a pale brown or chestnut-brown color. The fracture is conchoidal and glassy. It emits a somewhat peculiar nauseous odor by breathing on it. It has a very bitter taste and yields a greenish-yellow powder. It is partially soluble in cold water, leaving a soft resin undissolved. With hot water it gives a turbid, and with alcohol almost a clear solution.

Alumen.

[Alum]. Alaun.

[Sulphate of Aluminium and Potassium].

In more or less transparent, colorless, octohedral, hard, and slightly efflorescent crystals; soluble in about fifteen parts of cold water, and in equal parts of boiling water; insoluble in alcohol. A solution in water gives an acid reaction, and is not affected by hydrosulphuric acid. A diluted solution must not assume a bluish tint, immediately, on the addition of ferrocyanide of potassium, but only after some time. Alum, when heated with solution of caustic soda, should evolve no ammonia, and the primarily induced precipitate should be entirely soluble in an excess of the soda solution, and the liquid formed must scarcely be rendered turbid on the addition of hydrosulphate of ammonium.

Alumen ustum.

[BURNT ALUM]. Gebrannter Alaun.

Alum is calcined in a sufficiently capacious vessel of unglazed clay, until it is wholly converted into a light, spongy mass.

It is white, porous, easily pulverized, and has an acid reaction; it dissolves quite slowly, but almost wholly in water.

Alumina hydrata.

[HYDRATE OF ALUMINA]. Thonerdehydrat.

Argilla pura s. hydrata.

Take of Alum *ten parts*. 10

Dissolve it in

Warm Distilled Water *eighty parts*. . . . 80

Then filter, and add gradually, while stirring constantly, of

Pure Carbonate of Sodium *nine parts*, . . 9

dissolved in

Distilled Water *eighty parts*. 80

Let the precipitate subside, and, having poured off the supernatant liquid, collect it on a filter, and wash with water until the washings scarcely become turbid with nitrate of barium. The precipitate is expressed between bibulous paper, dried, and reduced to a very fine powder.

It is a white, light powder, adhering to the tongue; insoluble in water, but wholly soluble in diluted acids, and in solution of caustic soda; the alkaline solution is precipitated by chloride of ammonium, but it does not become turbid with hydrosulphate of ammonium, and, after the addition of hydrochloric acid in slight excess, is rendered only slightly cloudy with chloride of barium.

Ammoniacum.

[AMMONIAC. GUM AMMONIAC]. Ammoniakgummi.

Gummi-resina ammoniacum.

Dorema ammoniacum *Don.*

In roundish tears, from the size of a pea to that of a walnut, either embedded in a brownish mass, or agglutinated irregularly together in a lump; of a yellow or a yellowish-brown color externally. The fracture is slightly conchoidal, milk-white, and of a waxy lustre; translucent at the edges; rather hard when cold, becoming soft by heat. It irritates the fauces, when chewed, having a bitter taste and peculiar odor; it yields a milky fluid when triturated with water, and is but partially soluble in alcohol.

Brown gum ammoniac, intermixed with much impurity, should be rejected. For pharmaceutical purposes it is exposed to frost, then reduced to powder, and separated from impurities by means of a sieve.

Ammonium carbonicum.

[CARBONATE OF AMMONIUM]. Flüchtiges Laugensalz.

Sal volatile siccum. Ammoniacum carbonicum. Reines Hirschhornsalz.

In dense, hard, fibro-crystalline, translucent and dry masses, of a strongly ammoniacal, but no empyreumatic, odor. It effloresces in the air, and is often covered with a white powder. It is completely soluble in four parts of cold water, but dissolves with some difficulty in alcohol. It effervesces with acids, and is wholly volatilized by a moderate heat.

An aqueous solution, saturated with nitric acid, is not rendered turbid by hydrosulphuric acid, chloride of barium, or oxalate of ammonium; and nitrate of silver produces only a very slight cloudiness.

It should be preserved in very tightly-closed vessels.

Ammonium carbonicum pyro-oleosum.

[PYRO-CARBONATE OF AMMONIUM]. Brenzlich-kohlensaures Ammonium.

Ammoniacum carbonicum pyro-oleosum. Sal volatile cornu cervi.

Take of Carbonate of Ammonium *thirty-two parts*. . 32
Triturate it intimately into a powder with
Ethereal Animal Oil *one part*, ... 1
which is added gradually by drops.

It forms a whitish powder, which turns to a yellowish color by age. With water it yields a yellowish solution.

It should be preserved in a well-closed glass vessel.

Ammonium chloratum.

[CHLORIDE OF AMMONIUM]. Salmiak.

[Sal Ammoniac]. Ammoniacum hydrochloratum. Sal ammoniacum depuratum.

In white, hard, fibro-crystalline cakes, or in a white crystalline powder; colorless and inodorous, permanent in the air, and wholly volatilized by heat; soluble in three parts of cold water, and in an equal part of boiling water.

The aqueous solution is not altered by hydrosulphuric acid, hydrosulphate of ammonium, or chloride of barium. Ferrocyanide of potassium, dropped into a moderately dilute solution, produces only after some time a blue color.

Ammonium chloratum ferratum.

[AMMONIO-CHLORIDE OF IRON]. Eisensalmiak.

Ammoniacum hydrochloratum ferratum. Ammonium muriaticum martiatum.

Take of Chloride of Ammonium *sixteen parts*. . . 16
Dissolve it in
Distilled Water *thirty-two parts*, . . . 32
and add of
Solution of Sesquichloride of Iron *three parts*. . 3

Then evaporate the liquid to dryness in a porcelain capsule, by means of a steam-bath, stirring constantly, and reduce the remaining mass to a powder.

It forms an orange-yellow powder, deliquescent in the air, and wholly soluble in water. It contains 2.5 per cent. of iron, or 7.25 per cent. of sesquichloride of iron.

It should be preserved in well-closed vessels, in a dark place.

Ammonium phosphoricum.

[PHOSPHATE OF AMMONIUM]. Phosphorsaures Ammonium.

In colorless, transparent crystals, or in a white crystalline powder. It dissolves readily in water, but is insoluble in alcohol; it is neutral or but slightly alkaline.

An aqueous solution must not be affected by hydrosulphate of ammonium, nor, after being acidulated with hydrochloric acid, by hydrosulphuric acid, nor become turbid with chloride of barium.

Amygdalæ amaræ.

[BITTER ALMONDS]. Bittere Mandeln.

Semen amygdali amarum.

Amygdalus communis *Linn.* *a.* amara *D C.*

Oblong-ovate, somewhat compressed seeds; covered with a yellowish-brown, powdery skin (testa), which incloses a white, fleshy, oleaginous embryo, separable into two cotyledons; of a bitter taste, nearly inodorous, but diffusing a peculiar odor when triturated with water.

Old, rancid, or worm-eaten almonds are to be rejected.

Amygdalæ dulces.

[SWEET ALMONDS]. Süsse Mandeln.

Semen amygdali dulce.

Amygdalus communis *Linn.* *β.* dulcis *D C.*

The seeds are similar to the bitter almonds, generally larger and flatter, of a sweetish, oily taste; affording no odor when triturated with water.

Old, rancid, or worm-eaten almonds are to be rejected.

Amylum marantæ.

[ARROW-ROOT]. Marantastärke.

[***Maranta***].

Maranta arundinacea *Linn.*

A very fine, white, opaque, tasteless, and inodorous powder; insoluble in cold water and alcohol, giving with ninety-six parts of boiling water a moderately thin, pellucid mucilage, which, on the addition of iodine, assumes a violet-blue color. When arrow-root is shaken for ten minutes, with ten parts of a mixture—consisting of two parts of hydrochloric acid and one part of water—the greater part should separate unchanged, and it should not become mucilaginous, nor yield an herbaceous odor similar to that of green, unripe bean-pods.

Under the same name, not unfrequently, occur in commerce, the fecula of *Curcuma leucorrhiza* and *angustifolia* Roxb., from Malabar, and the fecula of *Manihot utilissima* Pohl., from Brazil. A compound microscope will easily show the difference of the granules. In Maranta arrow-root they are egg-shaped or oval, exhibiting well-marked layers, arranged (concentrically) one above the other, and at their broader end, each one shows a transverse fissure, or commonly a small eccentric nucleus. Curcuma fecula consists of flattened, ovate, or oblong-ovate granules; the one end of which is obtuse, the other end is more or less pointed, and provided with a very eccentrically situated point, or nucleus, surrounded by innumerable, very delicate, semilunar layers. The Manihot fecula consists, originally, of two, three, or four adherent granules, which separate on drying, each one exhibiting a kettledrum-shaped form, provided with a central point and concentric layers.

Care should be taken that it be not adulterated with potato starch, which yields, by the above given reaction, a thick mucilage, of the odor of green, unripe beans. The granules appear, under the compound microscope, more or less egg-shaped; one end obtuse, and the other considerably pointed, on which is exhibited an eccentrically situated point, around which run irregular concentric layers.

Amylum Tritici.

[WHEAT STARCH]. Weizenstärke.

Triticum vulgare ***Villars.***

A commercial article in irregular, angular masses, which yield, on being rubbed, a very fine, bluish-white, opaque powder without smell and taste, insoluble in cold water and alcohol. Under the compound microscope it appears to consist of lentil or nearly kidney-shaped disks, differing very much in size, having central points and obscurely marked concentric layers.

Wheat starch yields with ninety-six parts of boiling water a somewhat milky-white mucilage, which is colored violet-blue on the addition of iodine. When shaken with ten parts of a mixture consisting of two parts of hydrochloric acid and one part of water, it forms an inodorous mucilage.

Antidotum Arsenici.

[ANTIDOTE TO ARSENIOUS ACID]. Gegengift der arsenigen Säure.

Take of Solution of Persulphate of Iron *sixty parts*, . 60
Common Water *one hundred and twenty parts*. . 120

Mix, and add of
Calcined Magnesia *seven parts*, ... 7

previously triturated, intimately, with
Common Water *one hundred and twenty parts*, . 120

then shake together constantly, until a soft homogeneous pulp is produced.

It is prepared only when wanted for dispensing. There should be kept ready on hand, about 500 grammes of solution of persulphate of iron, and 150 grammes of calcined magnesia.

Aquæ destillatæ.

[DISTILLED WATERS]. Destillirte Wässer.

The distilled waters should possess, with the exception of opium water, the peculiar odor and taste of the substances from which they are prepared. They must be freed from the undissolved essential oils. Mucilaginous, and colored waters should be rejected.

They must be preserved in a cool place.

Aqua Amygdalarum amararum.

[BITTER ALMOND WATER]. Bittermandelwasser.

Aqua Amygdalarum amararum concentrata.

Take of Bitter Almonds *twelve parts*. 12

Bruise them, and express the fixed oil as much as possible, by means of a press, without the aid of heat. Reduce the mass to a fine powder and mix it thoroughly with

Common Water *eighty parts*, ... 80

then add, of

Alcohol *two parts*, ... 2

and distill off *ten parts*, ... 10

or so much, that *one thousand parts* of the well-mixed distillate contain *one part* of hydrocyanic acid, or that *one thousand parts*, being first treated with ammonio-nitrate of silver, and then with nitric acid, yield *five parts* of dry cyanide of silver.

Bitter Almond Water is somewhat cloudy, and has a strong odor of hydrocyanic acid and oil of bitter almonds. The odor of bitter almond oil must remain after the removal of hydrocyanic acid by means of nitrate of silver.

It should be *cautiously* preserved in well-closed bottles.

Aqua amygdalarum amararum diluta.

[DILUTED BITTER ALMOND WATER]. Kirschwasser.

[Cherry Water]. Aqua cerasorum. Aqua cerasorum amygdalata.

Take of Bitter Almond Water *one part*, ... 1

Distilled Water *nineteen parts*. 19

Mix them.

Aqua aromatica.

[AROMATIC WATER]. Schlagwasser.

Aqua cephalica. Aqua s. Balsamum Embryonum.

Take of Sage Leaves *four parts*, ...	4
Rosemary Leaves, ...	2
Peppermint, ...	2
Lavender Flowers, each, *two parts*, ...	2
Fennel Seed, ...	1
Cassia Bark, each, *one part*, ...	1
Alcohol *twenty-six parts*, ...	26
Common Water *one hundred and thirty parts*. .	130

Let the cut and bruised ingredients macerate for twenty-four hours, then distill off *seventy-two parts*. . 72

It should have a strongly aromatic odor. It is turbid.

Aqua calcariæ.

[LIME WATER]. Kalkwasser.

Aqua calcariæ ustæ. Aqua calcis. Calcaria soluta.

Take of Burnt Lime *one part*, ... 1

Having been slaked with a sufficient quantity of water, mix it, under brisk agitation, with

Common Water *fifty parts*. 50

Set aside for a few hours, stirring occasionally, and then pour off the liquid, from the greater part of the sediment, into a vessel furnished with a tightly-fitting stopper. It should be filtered before dispensing.

It is clear and colorless after filtration. It has an alkaline reaction, becomes turbid by heat and by blowing into it the air of the lungs.

Aqua chamomillæ.

[CHAMOMILE WATER]. Kamillenwasser.

Take of German Chamomile Flowers *one part*, . . . 1
Common Water *a sufficient quantity*.

Distill off *ten parts*. 10

Or it may be prepared by mixing
Concentrated Chamomile Water *one part*, . . 1
Distilled Water *nine parts*. 9

Aqua chamomillæ concentrata.

[CONCENTRATED CHAMOMILE WATER]. Koncentrirtes Kamillenwasser.

Take of German Chamomile Flowers *ten parts.* . . 10
Distill off by means of steam *one hundred parts.* . 100
Mix with the distillate
Alcohol *two parts,* 2
and again distill *ten parts.* 10
It should be preserved in stopped glass bottles.

Aqua chlorata.

[CHLORINE WATER]. Chlorwasser.

Aqua chlori. Chlorum solutum. Liquor Chlori. Aqua oxymuriatica.

A clear, yellowish-green liquid, of a suffocating odor. It instantly discolors blue litmus paper.

When shaken with so much metallic mercury, that the chlorine be entirely absorbed, the remaining liquid must not redden blue test-paper, or only in a very small degree.

One hundred parts of chlorine water, when shaken with *three parts* of crystallized protosulphate of iron, previously dissolved in water, acidulated with hydrochloric acid, must no longer discolor a solution of permanganate of potassium. It contains therefore nearly 0.4 per cent. of chlorine.

It must be protected from the light, and always kept in small, completely filled, glass-stoppered bottles.

Aqua cinnamomi.

[CINNAMON WATER]. Einfaches Zimmtwasser.

Take of Cassia Bark *one part,* 1
Common Water *a sufficient quantity.*
Distill off *ten parts.* 10

Aqua cinnamomi spirituosa.

[SPIRITUOUS CINNAMON WATER]. Weingeistiges Zimmtwasser.

Aqua cinnamomi vinosa.

Take of Cassia Bark *one part*, ... 1
Diluted Alcohol *one part*, ... 1
Common Water *ten parts*. 10
Distill off *five parts*. 5
It is turbid at first, and afterwards becomes clear.

Aqua communis.

[COMMON WATER. WATER]. Gemeines Wasser. Wasser.

The purest that can be had should be used; either well, river, or rain water.

When it cannot be had colorless, clear, and free from bad taste, it should be filtered through alternate layers of sand and charcoal.

Aqua destillata.

[DISTILLED WATER]. Destillirtes Wasser.

It should contain no foreign substances, excepting very small traces of carbonic acid or ammonia.

Aqua florum aurantii.

[ORANGE-FLOWER WATER]. Orangenblüthenwasser.

Aqua florum naphæ.

Take of Commercial Orange-Flower Water,
Distilled Water, *equal parts*.

Mix them.
It should be free from metallic impurities.

Aqua fœniculi.

[FENNEL WATER]. Fenchelwasser.

Take of Fennel Seed, bruised, *one part*, ... 1
Common Water *a sufficient quantity*.
Distill off *thirty parts*. 30

Fennel Water is somewhat turbid.

Aqua fœtida antihysterica.

[COMPOUND ASSAFETIDA WATER]. Zusammengesetztes Stinkasantwasser.

Aqua Asæ fœtida composita. Aqua fœtida Pragensis. Aqua antihysterica Pragensis.

Take of Galbanum *eight parts*, ... 8
Assafetida *twelve parts*, ... 12
Myrrh *six parts*, ... 6
Valerian Root, ... 16
Zedoary Root, each, *sixteen parts*, . . . 16
Angelica Root *four parts*, ... 4
Peppermint *twelve parts*, ... 12
Wild Thyme (Thymus Serpyllum), . . . 8
Roman Chamomile, each, *eight parts*, . . 8
Canada Castor *one part*. 1

Cut and bruise the ingredients, introduce them into a retort, and add of
Diluted Alcohol *one hundred and fifty parts*. . 150
Set the mixture aside for twenty-four hours, then add of
Common Water *three hundred parts*, ... 300
and distill off *three hundred parts*. 300
Compound Assafetida Water is turbid.

Aqua Kreosoti.

[CREASOTE WATER]. Kreosotwasser.

Kreosotum solutum.

Take of Creasote *one part*, ... 1
Distilled Water *one hundred parts*. 100

Mix by shaking.
Creasote Water is turbid.

Aqua Lauro-Cerasi.

[CHERRY-LAUREL WATER]. Kirschlorbeerwasser.

Take of Fresh Cherry-Laurel Leaves *twelve parts*. . 12
They are cut, and by means of a wooden pestle, bruised in a stone mortar, and, having poured upon them
Common Water *thirty-six parts*, ... 36
Alcohol *one part*, ... 1
distill into a well-cooled receiver *ten parts*, ... 10
or as much as will produce a water equal in strength to bitter almond water.

Cherry-laurel water is clear or nearly so, having the penetrating odor of hydrocyanic acid.

It should be *cautiously* preserved in well-closed bottles.

Aqua Melissæ.

[Balm Water. Melissa Water]. Melissenwasser.

Aqua Melissæ citratæ.

It is prepared from Balm Leaves, or from Concentrated Balm Water, like Chamomile Water.

It should be clear.

Aqua Melissæ concentrata.

[Concentrated Balm Water]. Koncentrirtes Melissenwasser.

It is prepared from Balm Leaves, like Concentrated Chamomile Water.

Aqua Menthæ crispæ.

[Curled-mint Water]. Krauseminzwasser.

Take of Curled-mint (Mentha Crispa) *one part*, . . . 1
Common Water *a sufficient quantity.*

Distill off *ten parts*. 10

It is slightly turbid.

Aqua Menthæ piperitæ.

[Peppermint Water]. Pfefferminzwasser.

It is prepared from Peppermint, like Curled-mint Water.

Peppermint Water is slightly turbid.

Aqua Menthæ piperitæ spirituosa.

[Spirituous Peppermint Water]. Weingeistiges Pfefferminzwasser.

Aqua menthæ piperitæ vinosa.

It is prepared from Peppermint, like Spirituous Cinnamon Water.

It is turbid.

Aqua Opii.

[Opium Water]. Opiumwasser.

Take of Opium, coarsely powdered, *one part*, . . 1
Common Water *ten parts*. 10
Distill off *five parts*. 5

Opium Water should be clear and colorless. It has a faint odor.

Aqua Petroselini.

[Parsley Water]. Petersilienwasser.

Take of Parsley Seed *one part*, ... 1
Common Water *a sufficient quantity*.
Distill off *twenty parts*. 20

It is slightly turbid at first, and afterwards becomes clear.

Aqua phagedænica.

[Phagedenic Water]. Phagedänisches Wasser.

[*Yellow Wash*]. ***Altschadenwasser. Liquor Hydrargyri bichlorati corrosivi cum Calcaria usta.***

Take of Corrosive Chloride of Mercury *one part*. . . 1
Powder it very finely, and mix with
Lime Water *three hundred parts*. . . . 300

It is turbid and yields an orange-yellow precipitate.
It is prepared only when wanted for dispensing.

Aqua phagedænica nigra.

[Black Wash]. Schwarzes Wasser.

Aqua Nigra. Aqua mercurialis nigra. Liquor Hydrargyri chlorati mitis cum Calcaria usta.

Take of Mild Chloride of Mercury *one part*, . . . 1
Lime Water *sixty parts*. 60
Mix by rubbing them well together.

The liquor is shaken up and dispensed with its black precipitate.

It is prepared only when wanted for dispensing.

Aqua Picis.

[TAR WATER]. Theerwasser.

Aqua picea.

Take of Tar *one part*. 1
Pour upon it
Hot Distilled Water *ten parts*. 10

Macerate for two days, stirring frequently, then pour off the clear liquid.

Tar Water is clear, somewhat yellowish, and possesses the odor and taste of tar.

It should be preserved in well-closed vessels.

Aqua Plumbi.

[LEAD WATER]. Bleiwasser.

Kühlwasser. Aqua plumbica s. saturnina.

Take of Distilled Water *forty-nine parts*, ... 49
Solution of Subacetate of Lead *one part*. . . 1

Mix them.

Lead Water is slightly turbid. Before dispensing it is shaken up.

It should be *cautiously* preserved.

Aqua Plumbi Goulardi.

[GOULARD'S LEAD WATER]. Goulard's Bleiwasser.

Aqua Goulardi. Aqua vegeto-mineralis Goulardi. Aqua Plumbi spirituosa.

Take of Common Water *forty-five parts*, ... 45
Solution of Subacetate of Lead *one part*, . . 1
Diluted Alcohol *four parts*. 4

Mix them.

It is turbid. Before dispensing it is shaken up.

It should be *cautiously* preserved.

Aqua Rosæ.

[Rose Water]. Rosenwasser.

Take of Fresh Rose Leaves *two parts*. 2
Or of such as are preserved with one-half part of chloride of sodium *three parts*, ... 3
Common Water *a sufficient quantity*.
Distill off *ten parts*. 10
Rose Water is clear.

Aqua Rubi Idæi.

[Raspberry Water]. Himbeerwasser.

Take of Fresh, Expressed Cakes of Raspberries *one hundred parts*, ... 100
Common Water *a sufficient quantity*.
Distill off *two hundred parts*. 200
Or it may be prepared by mixing
Concentrated Raspberry Water *one part*, . . 1
Distilled Water *nine parts*. 9

Aqua Rubi Idæi concentrata.

[Concentrated Raspberry Water]. Koncentrirtes Himbeerwasser.

Take of Fresh, Expressed Cakes of Raspberries *one hundred parts*, ... 100
Alcohol *four parts*, ... 4
Common Warm Water *a sufficient quantity*.
Macerate for one night, then distill off *twenty parts*. . 20
It is clear.
It should be preserved in well-closed vessels.

Aqua Salviæ.

[Sage Water]. Salbeiwasser.

It is prepared from Sage Leaves, or Concentrated Sage Water, like Chamomile Water.

It is somewhat cloudy at first, and afterwards becomes clear.

Aqua Salviæ concentrata.

[CONCENTRATED SAGE WATER]. Koncentrirtes Salbeiwasser.

It is prepared from Sage Leaves, like Concentrated Chamomile Water.

Aqua Sambuci.

[ELDER FLOWER WATER]. Fliederblumenwasser.

Hollunderblüthenwasser.

It is prepared from Elder Flowers, or from Concentrated Elder Flower Water, like Chamomile Water.
It is somewhat cloudy.

Aqua Sambuci concentrata.

[CONCENTRATED ELDER FLOWER WATER]. Koncentrirtes Fliederblumenwasser.

It is prepared from Elder Flowers, like Concentrated Chamomile Water.

Aqua Tiliæ.

[LINDEN FLOWER WATER]. Lindenblüthenwasser.

It is prepared from Linden Flowers, or Concentrated Linden Flower Water, like Chamomile Water.
It should be clear.

Aqua Tiliæ concentrata.

[CONCENTRATED LINDEN FLOWER WATER]. Koncentrirtes Lindenblüthenwasser.

It is prepared from Linden Flowers, like Concentrated Chamomile Water.

Aqua Valerianæ.

[VALERIAN WATER]. Baldrianwasser.

It is prepared from Valerian Root, like Curled-mint Water.
It should be clear, and redden blue test-paper.

Aqua vulneraria spirituosa.

[WHITE ARQUEBUSADE]. Weisse Arquebusade.

[Spirituous Vulnerary Water]. *Aqua vulneraria vinosa.*

Take of Peppermint,	1
Rosemary Leaves,	1
Rue Leaves,	1
Sage Leaves,	1
Wormwood,	1
Lavender Flowers, each, *one part.*	1
Cut them and macerate for two days in	
Diluted Alcohol *eighteen parts,*	18
Common Water *fifty parts.*	50
Then draw off by distillation *thirty-six parts.*	36

It is cloudy, and of a strongly aromatic odor.

Argentum foliatum.

[SILVER LEAF]. Blattsilber.

It should be as free as possible from other metals.

Argentum nitricum crystallisatum.

[CRYSTALLIZED NITRATE OF SILVER]. Krystallisirtes salpetersaures Silberoxyd.

In colorless, four or six-sided plates; permanent in the air; wholly soluble in water, alcohol, and ether. They form a colorless solution with water of ammonia. When heated on charcoal, with the blowpipe, they first melt, then deflagrate, and are finally converted into a globule of pure silver.

The aqueous solution, after the complete precipitation of silver, by means of hydrochloric acid, then filtered and evaporated, must yield no residue.

It should be *cautiously* preserved in a blackened, well-stopped bottle.

Argentum nitricum fusum.

[FUSED NITRATE OF SILVER]. Geschmolzenes salpetersaures Silberoxyd.

[*Lunar Caustic*]. ***Höllenstein. Lapis infernalis.***

It is white or grayish-white, solid, and exhibits a radiated fracture. It is completely soluble in ten parts of alcohol. With water of ammonia it forms a perfectly colorless solution. It has the chemical properties of crystallized nitrate of silver.

It should be *cautiously* preserved in a blackened, well-stopped bottle.

Argentum nitricum cum Kali nitrico.

[NITRATED LUNAR CAUSTIC]. Salpeterhaltiger Höllenstein.

Argentum nitricum fusum mitigatum.

Lapis infernalis nitratus.

Take of Crystallized Nitrate of Silver *one part*, . . . 1
Nitrate of Potassium *two parts*. 2

Mix by rubbing them together; melt the mixture in a porcelain vessel, and pour it into proper moulds.

In white, solid sticks, showing scarcely a crystalline fracture. *One hundred parts*, dissolved in water and mixed with hydrochloric acid in large excess, should yield no less than *twenty-seven parts*, well dried, chloride of silver.

It should be *cautiously* preserved in a blackened, well-stopped bottle.

Argilla.

[ALUMINA]. Thon.

[***White Bole***]. ***Weisser Bolus. Bolus alba.***

A whitish, cohesive, friable earth, tenacious when moist, but it disintegrates in water; consisting principally of pure alumina.

When hydrochloric acid is poured upon it, but very little effervescence should be produced.* It should be free from sand.

---

* Dr. Buchner, in his German translation, says: "It effervesces but very little with hydrochloric acid," and Dr. Hager, in his, says: "It must not effervesce at all." Latin text—"Acido hydrochlorico affuso *minime* efferveseat."

Asa fœtida.

[ASSAFETIDA]. Stinkasant.

Gummi-resina Asa fœtida. Teufelsdreck.

Scorodosma fœtidum *Bunge*. **Ferula Asa fœtida** *Linn.*

In separate, or more or less conglutinated tears, or in irregular masses. The surface of freshly broken pieces is whitish, opaline, with a waxy lustre, assuming a purplish color in a short time, and ultimately changing to a dirty brown. Assafetida becomes sticky between the fingers, and has a very disagreeable, garlicky odor, and an unpleasant taste. When triturated with water, it produces a gray emulsion; it is but partially soluble in alcohol. Dark masses, and those containing stones and other impurities, should be rejected.

Assafetida should be powdered during frosty weather, and separated from impurities by means of a sieve.

Atropinum.

[ATROPIA]. Atropin.

A crystalline, yellowish-white powder, of a peculiar taste and alkaline reaction; soluble in about three hundred parts of cold water, more readily in boiling water, and in alcohol. It yields with concentrated sulphuric acid a colorless solution, which, after some time, becomes yellowish; with nitric acid it forms a yellowish, and ultimately a colorless solution. When placed on a platinum foil, and exposed to heat, it emits a white vapor, of a peculiar odor, and is wholly dissipated.

Even a highly diluted solution of Atropia will dilate the pupil of the eye.

It should be *very cautiously* preserved.

Atropinum sulfuricum.

[SULPHATE OF ATROPIA]. Schwefelsaures Atropin.

A crystalline, white, neutral powder, of a bitter taste, readily soluble in water, and alcohol. One part, dissolved in one thousand parts of water, has a bitter, nauseous taste, and dilates the pupil of the eye.

When exposed to heat on a platinum foil, it is decomposed, and wholly dissipated, while emitting an acrid vapor. It gives in general the reaction of Atropia.

It should be *very cautiously* preserved.

Auro-Natrium chloratum.

[CHLORIDE OF GOLD AND SODIUM]. Chlorgoldnatrium.

Aurum chloratum s. muriaticum natronatum.

Take of Pure Gold *sixty-five parts.* 65
Dissolve it in
Nitro-muriatic Acid *two hundred and sixty parts.* 260
Evaporate the solution, by the heat of a steam-bath, until a small quantity, taken out, solidifies on cooling.
Then add of
Chloride of Sodium, in powder, *one hundred parts,* 100
and, while stirring constantly, reduce to a dry state by means of the steam-bath.

It forms an orange-yellow powder, slightly deliquescent in the air, wholly soluble in water. When it is fully washed with alcohol on a filter, there will be left a residue of nearly one-half, which is insoluble in the alcohol. It should contain *fifty per cent.* of chloride of gold ($Au\ Cl_3$).

Preserve it *cautiously* in glass-stoppered bottles.

Aurum foliatum.

[GOLD LEAF]. Blattgold.

It is insoluble in nitric acid. The nitric acid, having been in contact with the gold, must not become colored by the addition of water of ammonia in excess.

Balsamum Copaivæ.

[BALSAM OF COPAIBA]. Kopaivabalsam.

Copaifera multijuga *Hayne*, and other species of Copaifera.

A strongly odorous, pellucid, yellowish or brownish-yellow liquid, of the consistence of a fixed oil, having a somewhat bitter and acrid taste. When evaporated, it does not diffuse the odor of oil of turpentine, and it leaves a friable resin as a residue.

Balsamum Peruvianum.

[BALSAM OF PERU]. Perubalsam.

Balsamum Peruvianum nigrum. Balsamum Indicum.

Myroxylon Sonsonatense ***Klotzsch.***

A dark-brown liquid, showing a purplish-brown color in thin layers when viewed by transmitted light; it is greasy to the touch, non-drying in the air, of a syrupy consistence, and has an acid reaction; specific gravity of from 1.15 to 1.16; having a pleasant vanilla-like odor, and a somewhat bitter taste; producing a persistent acrid impression in the throat. It is almost wholly soluble in six parts of alcohol, forming a cloudy solution; it yields no essential oil by distillation in water.

One thousand parts of the balsam should neutralize seventy-five parts of crystallized carbonate of sodium.

It is not miscible with a large bulk of a fixed oil, but easily so with an essential oil. When mixed with an equal weight of concentrated sulphuric acid, it becomes heated, and, after cooling and washing it with water, hardens entirely into a compact mass, to which must adhere no fatty matter, occasioned by the admixture of balsam of copaiba or castor oil.

Balsamum Tolutanum.

[BALSAM OF TOLU]. Tolubalsam.

Balsamum de Tolu.

Myroxylon toluiferum ***Humboldt, Bonpland et Kunth*** (**Myrospermum toluiferum** ***Richard***).

A resinous mass; in the recent state it is soft, translucent, yellow or yellowish, of the consistence of (European) turpentine; by age it turns to a brownish color, and ultimately becomes quite brown, solid, and sometimes crystalline. It has a fragrant odor, and an aromatic, somewhat sweetish taste. It is soluble in acetone, alcohol, chloroform, and solution of caustic potassa, but insoluble in benzine, or bisulphide of carbon.

Baryum chloratum.

[CHLORIDE OF BARIUM]. Chlorbaryum.

Baryta muriatica.

In colorless, translucent, rhomboidal, tabular or lamellar crystals; permanent in the air; soluble in two and a half parts of cold water, and in one and a half parts of boiling water. The aqueous solution is colorless, and has no effect on test-paper; it is copiously precipitated by nitrate of silver, and diluted sulphuric acid, but it is not rendered turbid by hydrosulphate of ammonium, or hydrosulphuric acid.

Alcohol, shaken with the powdered crystals, must not take up a deliquescent salt, nor burn with a red flame.

Benzinum.

[BENZINE]. Benzin.

Benzinum Petrolei.

A transparent, colorless liquid, of a peculiar odor, produced in the distillation of American petroleum. It is very slightly soluble in water,* freely soluble in alcohol and ether; specific gravity of from 0.680 to 0.700; boils between 60° and 80° C., and is very inflammable. It should not be mixed with benzole, procured by the dry distillation of stone-coal, which is detected by the method used for testing petroleum-naphtha.

Benzoe.

[BENZOIN]. Benzoe.

Resina Benzoe.

Styrax Benzoin ***Dryander.*** (**Benzoin officinale** *Hayne*).

Either in agglutinated, shining tears, externally of a yellowish-brown or reddish-brown color, and internally milk-white; or in solid, reddish-brown masses, interspersed with paler tears. Benzoin has a very agreeable, vanilla-like odor.

Care should be taken that it be not adulterated with a resin, commonly called Penang or Sumatra Benzoin, which consists of numerous whitish, opaque pieces, imbedded in a scanty, pale-brown mass. Sumatra Benzoin has the odor of styrax, and, when boiled with milk of lime, on the addition of permanganate of potassium, exhales the odor of oil of bitter almonds.

---

* "Not at all soluble in water."—DR. HAGER, *Ger. Transl.*
"Very slightly soluble in water."—DR. BUCHNER, *Ger. Transl.*

Bismuthum subnitricum.

[SUBNITRATE OF BISMUTH]. Basisches salpetersaures Wismuthoxyd.

Bismuthum hydrico-nitricum. Magisterium Bismuthi.

Take of Pure Nitric Acid *nine parts.* 9
Introduce it into a glass retort, and add gradually of
Bismuth, coarsely powdered, *two parts,* . . 2

and facilitate the process of solution towards the end by a gentle heat. When nitrous fumes no longer escape, add Distilled Water, in amount equal to one-half of the solution, or until a white precipitate begins to fall. After the subsidence of the precipitate, decant and evaporate the supernatant liquid to the point of crystallization, or until it be three times the weight of the metal employed. Of the crystals, which have been washed with a small quantity of water, acidulated with a little nitric acid, and carefully triturated, take *one part,* mix it with *four parts* of Distilled Water, and pour the mixture into a vessel containing *twenty-one parts* of Hot Distilled Water, and stir briskly. Collect the resulting precipitate, immediately after cooling, on a filter, wash sparingly with water, and dry it at a temperature not exceeding 30° C.

It is a very white, crystalline powder, which, when moistened with water, reddens blue test-paper. It is dissolved by nitric or hydrochloric acid, without effervescence, forming a clear solution.

The solution formed by the action of nitric acid, and somewhat diluted with water, is not rendered turbid by nitrate of silver, nitrate of barium, or diluted sulphuric acid.

If the powder be boiled with ten times its weight of diluted acetic acid, and the solution wholly precipitated by hydrosulphuric acid and filtered; the filtrate should leave no residue when evaporated in a porcelain capsule. When heated with solution of caustic potassa, in excess, the resulting liquid should emit no ammonia, and, if then diluted with water, and filtered, should not become turbid with hydrosulphuric acid. To test it for arsenious acid: heat the preparation with an equal weight of concentrated sulphuric acid, until all nitric acid is dissipated; then dilute it with six times its quantity of water, and proceed as with pure hydrochloric acid.

It should be preserved in well-closed vessels.

Bismuthum valerianicum.

[VALERIANATE OF BISMUTH]. Baldriansaures Wismuthoxyd.

Take of Subnitrate of Bismuth *thirty-two parts*. . . 32

Rub it in a porcelain mortar with a small quantity of distilled water until it is reduced to a very soft pulp, then add it to a solution made with

Pure Carbonate of sodium *twelve parts*, . . 12
Distilled Water *thirty parts*, ... 30

previously mixed with

Valerianic Acid *nine parts*, ... 9

digest for an hour, at a gentle heat, stirring occasionally, then collect the precipitate on a filter upon cooling, wash with cold water, and dry it on a tile in a moderately warm place. It forms a white powder, having the odor of valerianic acid. It is insoluble in water, but soluble in hydrochloric acid, and in nitric acid. The solution produced by nitric acid is not rendered turbid by chloride of barium, or nitrate of silver. A gramme of the powder, repeatedly moistened with nitric acid, yields, on being exposed to heat, about 0.79 of a gramme of oxide of bismuth.

Borax.

[BORAX. BORATE OF SODIUM]. Borax.

[Biborate of Sodium]. Natrum biboricum s. biboracicum.

In white, hard, crystalline pieces, or prismatic crystals; soluble in from twelve to fifteen parts of cold water, and in two parts of boiling water, yielding a colorless solution, which turns yellow test-paper brown. The solution of borax is not affected by hydrosulphuric acid, or carbonate of sodium, nor, on being further diluted with water, rendered turbid by chloride of barium, or nitrate of silver. If a slight precipitate should be produced, it disappears on the addition of nitric acid.

Bromum.

[BROMINE]. Brom.

A blackish-red liquid, recognized by its sharp, peculiar chlorine-like odor. Its specific gravity is between 2.95 and 3.00. It boils between 58° and 63° C., and gives off, even at ordinary temperatures, yellowish-red fumes, affecting the eyes and lungs dangerously. It is soluble in thirty parts of water. Alcohol and ether dissolve bromine freely. It is entirely dissolved by solution of caustic soda; the resulting liquid, mixed with fuming nitric acid, in slight excess, must not communicate a violet color to bisulphide of carbon when shaken together.

It should be *cautiously* preserved in a tightly-fitting, glass-stoppered bottle, which must be inclosed in another larger glass or metallic vessel.

Bulbus Scillæ.

[SQUILL]. Meerzwiebel.

Scilla maritima *Linn.* (**Urginea Scilla** *Steinheil*).

The inner scales of the bulb, cut in pieces, which, on drying, become horny in appearance; they are translucent, whitish, and have a mucilaginous, nauseous, bitter taste.

Brown, tough or moist scales should be rejected.

Cadmium sulfuricum.

[SULPHATE OF CADMIUM]. Schwefelsaures Kadmiumoxyd.

In colorless, transparent, prismatic crystals, efflorescent in the air, and readily soluble in water.

A solution in water, acidulated with a small quantity of hydrochloric acid, throws down a lemon-yellow precipitate on the addition of hydrosulphuric acid, which precipitate is not soluble in water of ammonia. After a complete precipitation, in this manner, the (supernatant) filtered liquid leaves no residue on evaporation.

It should be *cautiously* preserved in well-closed vessels.

Calcaria carbonica præcipitata.

[PRECIPITATED CARBONATE OF CALCIUM]. Präcipitirter Kohlensaurer Kalk.

[*Precipitated Carbonate of Lime*].

A white, crystalline powder, insoluble in water, wholly soluble, with effervescence, in diluted acetic acid, hydrochloric acid, or nitric acid.

When shaken with distilled water, the filtrate should exhibit but a slight cloudiness with nitrate of silver, and leave no residue on evaporation.

Calcaria chlorata.

[CHLORINATED LIME. CHLORIDE OF LIME]. Chlorkalk.

Calcaria hypochlorosa. Calx chlorata.

A white or grayish-white powder, of a moderately strong chlorine odor; but partially soluble in water, leaving a residue of hydrate of lime. With hydrochloric acid an abundance of chlorine gas is developed.

When one hundred parts of chloride of lime, triturated with water, are mixed with an aqueous solution, containing one hundred and ninety-six (196) parts of pure protosulphate of iron, and then gradually mixed and shaken with hydrochloric acid, a liquid is formed, which, when filtered, should contain no protoxide of iron, and give, therefore, no blue color with ferridcyanide of potassium. The chloride of lime, consequently, contains no less than *twenty-five* per cent. of active chlorine.

It should be preserved in well-closed vessels, protected from the light.

Calcaria phosphorica.

[PHOSPHATE OF CALCIUM. PHOSPHATE OF LIME].
Phosphorsaure Kalkerde.

Take of Native Carbonate of Lime *twenty parts*, . . 20
dissolve it in
Pure hydrochloric Acid, ... 50
Distilled Water, each, *fifty parts*, . . . 50
allow it to settle for several hours, pour off the clear liquid, and, if contaminated with iron, add of
Chloride of Lime *one part*, ... 1
which has been rubbed to a paste with water. Let the mixture digest for several hours, then add of
Water of Ammonia *about two parts*, ... 2
so that it be in slight excess. To the filtered liquid add, while stirring, of
Phosphate of Sodium *fifty parts*, ... 50
dissolved in
Distilled Water *three hundred parts*. 300

Collect the resulting precipitate, after several hours, on a filter, wash well with water, and dry it at a gentle heat.

It forms a light, dazzling white powder, insoluble in water; slightly soluble in water containing carbonic acid. It dissolves with difficulty, or but partially, in acetic acid, without effervescence, and wholly in nitric acid, also without the escape of gas; the latter solution is rendered but slightly turbid by nitrate of silver, but no cloudiness is produced with chloride of barium, and, after the addition of water of ammonia in excess, a white, but in no case colored, precipitate should be produced by hydrosulphate of ammonium.

Calcaria sulfurica usta.

[CALCINED GYPSUM]. Gebrannter Gyps.

[*Plaster of Paris*]. *Gypsum ustum.*

A white, amorphous powder; when made into a paste with half its weight of water, the mixture becomes solid in a few minutes.

It should be preserved in well-closed vessels.

Calcaria usta.

[BURNT LIME]. Gebrannter Kalk.

Calcaria. Calx viva.

A dense, white mass, which, when moistened with about half its weight of water, becomes strongly heated, and falls into a white powder; with a larger quantity of water it forms a thick paste. This paste should dissolve in dilute nitric acid, almost without effervescence, leaving only a small portion undissolved; and the solution, neutralized with water of ammonia, must not be affected, or but slightly so, by hydrosulphate of ammonium.

It should be preserved in well-closed vessels.

Camphora.

[CAMPHOR]. Kampfer.

Camphora officinarum *Nees.* (**Laurus Camphora** *Linn*).

In white, pellucid masses, which break in irregular, angular, lamellar pieces, having a shining appearance, and tough consistence; becoming friable when sprinkled with alcohol. Camphor occurs in commerce in circular cakes, convex above and concave on their lower surface. It has a peculiar, penetrating, fragrant odor, and leaves a cooling sensation on the tongue. When heated, it melts, volatilizes, and burns with a bright flame, producing a dense smoke. It is insoluble in water, freely soluble in alcohol, ether, acetic acid, and in the fixed and essential oils.

It should be preserved in well-closed vessels.

Cantharides.

[CANTHARIDES]. Spanische Fliegen.

[*Spanish Flies*]. *Canthariden.* *Muscæ Hispanicæ.*

Lytta vesicatoria *Fabricius.*

Shining, golden-green beetles (coleoptera), from one and a half to three centimetres in length, furnished with black, filiform antennæ; having an unpleasant odor.

They may be gathered in June and July, and should be quickly and thoroughly dried, and *cautiously* preserved in well-closed vessels.

Carbo animalis.

[ANIMAL CHARCOAL]. Thierkohle.

Fleischkohle. Carbo Carnis.

Veal, freed of its fat and cut in small pieces, with about one-third part of small bones, is roasted in a suitable covered vessel as long as inflammable vapors escape. The residue, when cold, is reduced to powder, and preserved in a closed glass vessel.

A brownish-black powder of little luster, and scarcely any empyreumatic odor, burning without flame when exposed to a red heat; partially soluble in hydrochloric acid; the resulting liquid, when filtered, on the addition of water of ammonia, yields a precipitate of phosphate of calcium.

Carbo pulveratus.

[PREPARED CHARCOAL]. Holzkohle.

Carbo præparatus.

Charcoal, made of light wood, is heated so long as it yields smoke and flame, and is then put into a closed vessel where the fire is extinguished. It is freed from ashes, and, while still warm, reduced to a very fine powder, which is immediately inclosed tightly in a vessel, in which it is preserved.

A black, dry, tasteless powder, which, when heated, burns without flame.

Carboneum sulfuratum.

[BISULPHIDE OF CARBON]. Schwefelkohlenstoff.

Alcohol sulfuris.

A colorless liquid, of high refracting power, having a strong, peculiar odor. It is scarcely soluble in water, freely in alcohol, ether and the oils; of the specific gravity 1.272. It boils at a temperature of 46° C., is very volatile, and when ignited, burns with a blue flame, producing carbonic and sulphurous acids.

It should not affect test-paper, moistened with water. A solution of acetate of lead, shaken with bisulphide of carbon, should not be colored.

It should be preserved in well-closed bottles, in a cold place.

Caricæ.

[Figs]. Feigen.

Fructus Caricæ. Fici.

Ficus Carica *Linn.*

Consisting of fleshy, pear-shaped receptacles, with umbilicated apex, and filled with innumerable, very small, stony fruits (seeds). Figs have an agreeable, sweet taste.

Large, very fleshy, and very sweet—commonly termed Smyrna figs—should be selected. Dry, dark and nearly tasteless, or sourish, harsh or worm-eaten figs should be rejected.

Carrageen.

[Irish Moss]. Irländisches Moos.

Perlmoos. Knorpeltang. Caragaheen. Fucus crispus.

Chondrus crispus *Lyngbye*; (**Fucus crispus** *Linn.*), **etc.**

A flat or curled dichotomous thallus, with linear or wedge-shaped lobes; when dried it is cartilaginous, and of a yellowish-white color. A decoction gelatinizes on cooling.

Caryophylli.

[Cloves]. Gewürznelken.

Caryophylli aromatici.

Caryophyllus aromaticus *Linn.*

The flower buds with a nearly four-cornered, cylindrical, glandular calyx tube; calyx four-parted, supporting a closed, nearly globular, caducous corolla, which incloses the sexual organs. Cloves have a brown color, and a very strong, aromatic odor, and when chewed produce a strong, burning sensation in the mouth.

Cloves should be heavy, of greater gravity than water, and, when pressed between the fingers, give out an essential oil. Sour, pale, and shriveled cloves should be rejected.

Castoreum Canadense.

[CANADA CASTOR] Canadisches Bibergeil.

Castoreum Anglicum vel Americanum.

Castor Americanus ***Cuvier.***

The sacs are similar to those of the Siberian Castor; furnished externally with closely attached, inseparable membranes, filled with a resinous, somewhat hard mass, having a shining fracture, and a weak odor.

Care should be taken that they be not confounded with factitious sacs, which consist of a resin, covered with a membrane.

Castoreum Sibiricum.

[SIBERIAN OR RUSSIAN CASTOR]. Sibirisches Bibergeil.

Castoreum Moscoviticum, Rossicum, Polonicum, Germanicum, Europæum.

Castor Fiber ***Linn.***

Consisting frequently of two, more or less connected, glabrous, obovate, dark-brown sacs; having two exterior, rather thick, easily separable membranes, and two interior, thinner, and laminated ones, which traverse the cavity containing the castor. Recent castor is a thick, yellowish-brown, somewhat unctuous mass; when dry it becomes brown, opaque, friable, and effervesces with acids; it has a strong, peculiar odor.

Catechu.

[CATECHU]. Katechu.

Pegu-Catechu. Terra Japonica.

Acacia Catechu ***Wildenow.***

In irregular masses, covered and interspersed with leaves; externally of a dark liver-color, and internally of a uniform, dark-brown; porous and shining; inodorous, and of a somewhat bitter and a very astringent taste; soluble, partially, in water, and wholly in alcohol.

The so-called *Gambir Catechu*, in cubic pieces, and of a dark-brown color, with a dull, yellowish, earthy fracture; or in masses, not colored uniformly, but partially liver-brown, and partially dark-brown, with a dark, dull, earthy fracture, is to be rejected. And also the Catechu which is prepared from the seeds of *Areca Catechu* Linn., which occurs in circular, flat cakes, dark-brown and shining internally, and strewn with rice chaff on the surface.

Cera alba.

[WHITE WAX]. Weisses Wachs.

In white, brittle pieces; translucent in thin laminæ; of the specific gravity 0.97, not melting under a temperature of 63° or 64° C., otherwise, having the properties of yellow wax.

Care should be taken that it be not adulterated with paraffin, stearic acid, Japan or vegetable wax, or other fatty substances.

Cera flava.

[YELLOW WAX]. Gelbes Wachs.

Cera citrina.

Apis mellifica *Linn.*

In a more or less yellowish mass, breaks with a granular surface, softens by the heat of the hand, of a peculiar honey-like odor, having the specific gravity 0.96, melting at a temperature of 62° or 63° C., soluble in twenty parts of ether at a temperature of 15° C.

When thrown upon red-hot coal, the wax should not emit vapors of a fatty odor. It is wholly soluble in oil of turpentine. Shaken with cold, diluted alcohol, the filtrate should leave no resin, when evaporated.

Ceratum Æruginis.

[GREEN CERATE]. Grünes Wachs.

Grünspancerat. Ceratum viride. Emplastrum viride.

Take of Yellow Wax *twelve parts*, ... 12
Burgundy Pitch *six parts*, ... 6
Turpentine* *four parts*. 4

Melt them at a gentle heat, strain and diligently mix with

Verdigris, finely powdered, *one part*. . . 1

Pour the partially-cooled mass into paper capsules.†

The cerate has a deep-green color.

---

* See *Terebinthina*.

† Small paper moulds, made by turning up the four edges of rectangular pieces of paper, to form the plaster in flat, square or rectangular cakes, which are sometimes cut into still smaller pieces after being removed.

Ceratum Cetacei.

[SPERMACETI CERATE]. Walrathcerat.

Emplastrum Spermatis Ceti. Ceratum labiale album.

Take of White Wax, ... 2
Spermaceti, each, *two parts*, ... 2
[Expressed] Oil of Almonds *three parts*. . . 3

Melt them at a gentle heat, and pour the mass into paper capsules, and when cold, cut it into square cakes.

It should be white and free from rancidity.

Ceratum Cetacei rubrum.

[RED LIP SALVE]. Rothe Lippenpomade.

Ceratum labiale rubrum.

Take of [Expressed] Oil of Almonds *ninety parts*, . . 90
Alkanet Root *four parts*. 4

Digest until the oil has assumed a bright color, then strain and add of

White Wax *sixty parts*, ... 60
Spermaceti *ten parts*. 10

Melt in a proper vessel, add of

Oil of Bergamot, ... 1
Oil of Lemon, each, *one part*, ... 1

and pour the mass into paper capsules.

It should be red and free from rancidity.

Ceratum Myristicæ.

[NUTMEG CERATE]. Muskatbalsam.

[Nutmeg Balsam]. Balsamum Nucistæ.

Take of Yellow Wax *one part*, ... 1
Olive Oil *two parts*, ... 2
Oil of Nutmeg *six parts*. 6

Melt and pour the mass into paper capsules.

The cerate should have an orange-yellow color, and an aromatic odor.

Ceratum Resinæ Pini.

[Yellow Cerate. Resin Cerate]. Gelbes Cerat.

Ceratum Picis. Ceratum Resinæ Burgundicæ. Ceratum s. Emplastrum citrinum.

Take of Yellow Wax *four parts*, ... 4
Burgundy Pitch *two parts*, ... 2
Suet, ... 1
Turpentine, each, *one part*. 1

Melt and pour the mass into paper capsules.

Resin Cerate is tenacious and of a yellow color.

Cerussa.

[White Lead]. Bleiweiss.

Plumbum carbonicum s. hydrico-carbonicum.

A very white, heavy mass, partially pulverulent, adhering to the fingers, insoluble in water, but wholly soluble with effervescence in diluted nitric or acetic acid.

The solution produced by diluted acetic acid, yields a brown precipitate with hydrosulphuric acid; the filtrate must not be rendered turbid by carbonate of sodium.

It should be *cautiously* preserved.

Cetaceum.

[Spermaceti]. Walrath.

Sperma Ceti.

Physeter macrocephalus *Linn*, and other species of Physeter.

In irregular, very white, glistening, semi-translucent, foliated masses, unctuous to the touch, of a feeble odor, and insipid taste; specific gravity of from 0.94 to 0.95, melting between 45° and 50° C., soluble in warm alcohol and ether.

Rancid or yellowish spermaceti should be rejected.

Cetaceum saccharatum.

[Saccharated Spermaceti]. Walrathzucker.

Präparirter Walrath. Cetaceum cum Saccharo. Cetaceum præparatum.

Take of Spermaceti *one part*, ... 1
Sugar, best white, powdered, *three parts*, . . . 3

Mix, and rub them carefully into a very fine powder.

Charta nitrata.

[SALTPETER-PAPER]. Salpeterpapier.

Take of Nitrate of Potassium *one part*, ... 1
dissolve it in
Distilled Water *four parts*. 4

Soak bibulous paper in the solution and then dry it.

Charta resinosa.

[ANTI-RHEUMATIC PAPER]. Gichtpapier.

Charta antirrheumatica s. antarthritica.

Take of Black Pitch, ... 6
Turpentine, each, *six parts*, ... 6
Yellow Wax, *four parts*, ... 4
Resin (Colophony) *ten parts*. 10

Melt them together at a gentle heat, strain carefully, and spread the mass on paper.

It forms a brown, shining, adhesive plaster.

Chininum.

[QUINIA]. Chinin.

[***Quinine***].

An amorphous, white, very bitter powder, of an alkaline reaction, soluble in one thousand and two hundred parts of cold water, in two hundred and fifty parts of boiling water, more readily soluble in alcohol, less so in ether. When heated in water, it melts and attaches itself to the sides of the vessel. It is readily charred by heat and burns without residue. It dissolves easily in water, acidulated with sulphuric acid, which solution, though greatly diluted, is fluorescent. When this solution is mixed, first with chlorine water, and afterwards with water of ammonia in considerable excess, it changes to a green color.

Quinia or salts of quinia, treated with concentrated sulphuric acid, must not assume a red color. When heated with milk of lime, no ammoniacal odor should be evolved.

Dissolved in any diluted acid, on the addition of water of ammonia, it throws down a precipitate which disappears if ether be immediately added and the mixture shaken; and the liquid separates in two perfectly transparent layers.

Chinium bisulfuricum.

[BISULPHATE OF QUINIA]. Saures Schwefelsaures Chinin.

Chininum sulfuricum acidum.

In prismatic, white, shining crystals, of a very bitter taste, soluble in eight or ten parts of water, and in two parts of alcohol, giving an acid reaction.

It is tested like quinia to ascertain its purity.

Chininum ferro-citricum.

[CITRATE OF IRON AND QUINIA]. Citronensaures Eisen-Chinin.

Take of Citric Acid *six parts*, ... 6
dissolve it in
Distilled Water *one hundred parts*, . . . 100
and add of
Powdered Iron *three parts*, ... 3
which is dissolved at a gentle heat, and when no more hydrogen gas escapes, the solution is filtered. Evaporate the filtrate to one-fourth its weight and add of
Quinia *one part*, ... 1
and evaporate the liquid to the consistence of a syrup, and spread it, by means of a brush, on plates of glass or porcelain, and dry it in a moderately warm place.

It forms shining, transparent, reddish-brown scales, of a very bitter, ferruginous taste; readily soluble in water and and sparingly so in alcohol. An aqueous solution throws down a dark-blue precipitate on the addition both of ferrocyanide and ferridcyanide of potassium.

Chininum hydrochloricum.

[HYDROCHLORATE OF QUINIA. MURIATE OF QUINIA]. Salzsaures Chinin.

Chininum hydrochloratum s. muriaticum.

In white crystals of a silky lustre, frequently deposited in tufts; of a very bitter taste; soluble in about twenty parts of cold water, and in from two to three parts of alcohol.

A solution made with one part of the salt and one hundred parts of water, must not be rendered cloudy, in the least, by sulphuric acid, and but very slightly so by chloride of barium.

It is tested like quinia to ascertain its purity.

Chininum sulfuricum.

[SULPHATE OF QUINIA]. Schwefelsaures Chinin.

In snow-white, flexible and very tender, acicular crystals; of a silky lustre. Sulphate of quinia has a very bitter taste; it is soluble in about eight hundred parts of cold water, in thirty parts of boiling water, and in sixty parts of alcohol, and readily soluble in acidulated water, but of difficult solution in ether.

Twenty cubic centimetres of distilled water, at a temperature of 15° C., are poured upon two grammes of sulphate of quinia, in a cylindrical glass vessel, and thoroughly shaken, so that an emulsion-like liquid is produced. After a maceration of half an hour at a temperature of 15° C., the liquid is filtered. Five cubic centimetres of this filtrate are introduced into a test tube, and seven cubic centimetres of water of ammonia cautiously poured upon them, avoiding the mixing of the liquids as much as possible; if the tube be now closed with the finger and gently turned, there should be formed immediately, or after a short time, a perfectly clear liquid.

It is tested further like quinia to ascertain fully its purity.

It should be preserved in well-closed vessels.

Chininum tannicum.

[TANNATE OF QUINIA]. Gerbsaures Chinin.

Take of Sulphate of Quinia *one part*. 1
Dissolve it with a few drops of diluted sulphuric acid in
Distilled Water *thirty parts*, ... 30
and add gradually a solution, previously made, of
Tannic Acid *three parts*, ... 3
Cold Water *thirty parts*. 30

Let the precipitate subside in a cool place, collect it on a filter, wash with a small quantity of water, and dry it at a very gentle heat.

A yellowish, amorphous powder, of a peculiar odor and bitter, astringent taste. It dissolves sparingly in alcohol, and very sparingly in water. In hot water it melts into a mass.

Chininum valerianicum.

[VALERIANATE OF QUINIA]. Baldriansaures Chinin.

In white, shining crystals, of a very bitter taste, having a weak odor of valerianic acid; they are neutral to test-paper and dissolve in about one hundred parts of cold water, in forty parts of boiling water, and in six parts of alcohol; but dissolve with difficulty in ether. When dissolved in water and mixed with diluted sulphuric acid, the solution becomes fluorescent. The aqueous solution must not become turbid with chloride of barium, or but very slightly so.

It should be preserved in well-closed vessels.

Chinoidinum.

[QUINOIDIN. CHINOIDINE]. Chinoidin.

Chinioideum.

A brown or dark-brown, brittle, resinoid mass, having a conchoidal, shining fracture and a bitter taste; sparingly soluble in water, readily soluble in alcohol, and in diluted acids.

It yields, when rubbed with boiling-hot water, a colorless filtrate, which is not colored by solution of caustic potassa. It leaves but a very small quantity of ashes after incineration.

Chloralum hydratum crystallisatum.

[HYDRATE OF CHLORAL]. Krystallisirtes Chloralhydrat.

In dry, transparent, colorless crystals, having an aromatic odor, which, when the crystals are heated, becomes slightly pungent. The taste is somewhat bitter and slightly acrid; readily soluble in water, liberating no oily drops; also soluble in alcohol, ether, petroleum-naphtha, benzine, and in bisulphide of carbon. The crystals fuse at a temperature of from 56° to 58° C., and solidify at about 15° C.; they boil and are entirely volatilized at about 95° C.

Hydrate of Chloral, heated in solution of caustic potassa, renders the same cloudy, but the solution soon becomes clear on the separation of colorless chloroform. Heated with sulphuric acid, it is decomposed with the separation of chloral, but the liquid must not become brown. An aqueous solution is neutral to test paper, and, when acidulated with a little nitric acid, must not throw down a precipitate of chloride of silver, on the addition of nitrate of silver. It should not become moist in the air.

Preserve it in well-closed vessels.

Chloroformium.

[CHLOROFORM]. Chloroform.

Formylum trichloratum.

A transparent, colorless, and completely volatile liquid, specific gravity of from 1.492 to 1.496, having a peculiar odor and a sweetish taste; sparingly soluble in water, readily soluble in alcohol, ether, and the oils; boiling at a temperature of 61° or 62° C.

Distilled water shaken with chloroform, must not change blue test-paper, nor be rendered turbid by nitrate of silver. When chloroform is dropped into a solution of iodide of potassium, made with twenty times its weight of distilled water, the solution must not turn red.

It should be *cautiously* preserved in well-stopped, blackened, glass bottles.

Cinchoninum.

[CINCHONIA]. Cinchonin.

In white, often moderately thick, shining crystals, of an alkaline reaction. They have an indifferent taste at first, but afterwards peculiarly bitter; sparingly soluble in water, more freely in alcohol and chloroform; almost insoluble in ether. They are charred and then wholly dissipated by heat.

Cinchonia is freely soluble in diluted acids. The acidulous solutions show no fluorescence; if first treated with chlorine water, and then with water of ammonia in excess, they are not colored green; or, when shaken with water of ammonia, and then with ether, the resulting precipitate of cinchonia, is not redissolved.

Cinchoninum sulfuricum.

[SULPHATE OF CINCHONIA]. Schwefelsaures Cinchonin.

In white, hard, prismatic crystals, of a very bitter taste, soluble in about sixty parts of water, and in about seven parts of alcohol; insoluble in ether, readily soluble in acidulated water. The aqueous solution is slightly alkaline, otherwise it gives the same reactions as the salts of cinchonia.

Coccionella.

[COCHINEAL]. Cochenille.

Coccus Cacti ***Linn.***

In egg-shaped grains, flat or concave beneath, convex above, marked with transverse wrinkles. They are of a dark-purple or gray color, and are dusted with a white powder. They yield a dark-red powder, and impart a red color to alcohol.

The fraudulent admixture of lead may be detected when cochineal is triturated with water.

Codeinum.

[CODEIA]. Codein.

In white or yellowish-white, often clearly defined rhombic crystals, of an alkaline reaction and a bitter taste; when boiled in water they melt before dissolving; soluble in eighty parts of cold water, more readily soluble in alcohol, and ether; they dissolve in the same proportion in water of ammonia as in water; slightly soluble in solution of caustic potassa, and readily so in diluted acids. With concentrated sulphuric acid they yield a colorless solution, which turns blue on the addition of very little solution of sesquichloride of iron. Codeia is charred and then entirely dissipated by heat.

It should be *cautiously* preserved in well-closed bottles.

Coffeinum.

[CAFFEINE]. Kaffein.

[***Thein***]. ***Theinum.***

In colorless, soft, flexible, generally quite long and delicate crystals, of a silky lustre, having a bitter taste; soluble in about one hundred parts of cold water, in one hundred and sixty parts of absolute alcohol, and in three hundred parts of ether. They are dissolved freely in boiling water, so that a boiling saturated solution yields a soft crystalline mass upon cooling. When heated with chlorine water, or mixed with concentrated nitric acid, they are decomposed, and leave a yellow mass on being evaporated at a gentle heat, which, when moistened with water of ammonia, assumes a purplish-red color. They are completely volatilized by heat.

Colla piscium.

[ISINGLASS]. Hausenblase.

Ichthyocolla.

Acipenser Huso *Linn.*, and of other species of Acipenser.

In horny membranes, consisting either of leaves, or rolls twisted together in the form of a lyre; being tough and of a whitish color, transparent, iridescent, insipid, and inodorous; almost wholly soluble in boiling water, and boiling diluted alcohol. The solution, upon cooling, forms a gelatinous mass.

Yellow, brown, and less soluble isinglass should be rejected.

Collodium.

[COLLODION]. Collodium.

Take of Cotton *one part*, ... 1
Nitric Acid, of the specific gravity 1.420, *seven parts*, ... 7
Sulphuric Acid, of the specific gravity 1.833, *eight parts*, ... 8
or, if a nitric acid of that specific gravity is not on hand, take of
Nitric Acid, specific gravity of from 1.382 to 1.390, *eight parts*, ... 8
Sulphuric Acid, of the specific gravity 1.833, *twenty parts*. 20

The nitric and sulphuric acids are mixed, the mixture allowed to cool to the temperature of the air, the cotton is then introduced, so as to saturate it with the acids, and the whole is set aside from twelve to twenty-four hours. Then remove the compact mass, wash thoroughly with distilled water, express and dry it.

Agitate *one part* of this mass with a mixture of *eighteen parts* of Ether and *three parts* of Alcohol, and, after repose, pour off the clear liquid from the sediment.

Collodion is of a syrupy consistence, and should be preserved in well-stopped bottles.

Collodium cantharidatum.

[CANTHARIDAL COLLODION]. Blasenziehendes Collodium.

Collodium cantharidale. Collodium vesicans.

It is prepared like Collodion, but in place of ether, the Cantharidal Ether, *Æther cantharidatus*, is used, which is prepared in the following manner:

Take of Spanish Flies, in coarse powder, *four parts*, . 4
Ether *six parts*. 6
After due maceration, the filtrate should consist of *four parts*, ... 4
which should be preserved in a well-stopped bottle.

It forms a clear, brownish-green liquid.

Collodium elasticum.

[ELASTIC COLLODION]. Elastisches Collodium.

Collodium flexile.

Take of Collodion *fifty parts*, ... 50
Castor Oil *one part*. 1

Mix by agitation.

Colophonium.

[RESIN]. Geigenharz.

[*Colophony*]. ***Kolophonium. Resina Colophonium.***

A light yellow or yellowish-brown, translucent, brittle, very friable resin; exhibiting a broad and flat conchoidal fracture; nearly inodorous and tasteless, melting at a temperature of 135° C.; readily soluble in alcohol, ether, and in the fixed and essential oils.

Conchæ præparatæ.

[PREPARED OYSTER SHELLS]. Präparirte Austerschalen.

Oyster shells are boiled in common water, and cleaned from their impurities by means of a stiff brush, and are then well washed, dried, and reduced to an impalpable powder.

Prepared oyster shells form a white and very fine powder, which effervesces with hydrochloric acid; the resulting solution yields but a slight precipitate with water of ammonia.

Coniinum.

[CONIA. CONIINE]. Coniin.

A colorless or yellowish, oily liquid, of a peculiar, penetrating odor, having the specific gravity 0.89; miscible in all proportions with alcohol, ether, chloroform, and the oils. It is soluble in one hundred parts of cold water.

The aqueous solution has an alkaline reaction, becoming cloudy on warming, and regaining its limpidity on cooling. It is readily soluble in water, acidulated with hydrochloric acid, which solution must not yield a precipitate with bichloride of platinum. Conia does not become turbid when heated; it is entirely volatilized by heat.

It should be preserved *very cautiously* in well-closed vessels protected from the light.

Cortex Cascarillæ.

[CASCARILLA BARK]. Kaskarillrinde.

Croton Eluteria; Croton Cascarilla *Bennett.*

A compact bark, consisting of longitudinally curved, or quilled pieces, about two millimetres thick, having a thin periderm (corky layer), white externally, with intersected, furrowed fissures; this layer is often partially removed. The inner bark is a little thicker, also fissured on the outside, of a reddish-brown color and horny fracture; the cross section is marked with striated rays, collected in wedge-shaped bundles.

The bark when chewed produces a burning sensation in the mouth; it has a bitter taste and aromatic odor.

The intermixed branches are to be rejected.

Cortex Chinæ Calisayæ.

[CALISAYA BARK. YELLOW CINCHONA]. Kalisayarinde.

Königschina.* *Cortex Chinæ regius.

Cinchona Calisaya *Weddell.*

The liber (inner bark) of the trunk; it is flattish, of a reddish-yellow color, from one to two centimetres in thickness, showing on a transverse section, radially arranged bast-cells dissociated by the (intercellular) parenchyma; having, on the exterior surface, large, slightly conchoidal depressions with sharp margins, or being frequently covered, interruptedly, with hard, cortical scales, consisting of alternate pale and dark layers. It has a uniform fracture with very short and rigid fibres, and a smooth interior surface, which, owing to protuding cellular fibres, has a shining appearance.

The preference is given to the so-called Bolivian Monopoly-Bark. Calisaya Bark should not be confounded with the yellow or red *Pitaya* bark, which is brought from New Grenada. It should contain no less than two per cent. of cinchona alkaloids.

Cortex Chinæ fuscus.

[BROWN CINCHONA*]. Braune Chinarinde.

[***Pale Bark.* *Gray Bark*].** ***China grisea.***

Cinchona micrantha *Ruiz et Pavon*, and of other species of Cinchona.

The bark of the branches, nearly three millimetres in thickness, consisting of quills from the size of a goosequill to that of the little finger, having in the middle layer a nearly black, resinous circle; the fracture is smooth towards the exterior surface, and fibrous inwardly.

The *Huanuco* bark, of a cinnamon color, exhibiting white patches on the outer surface with numerous, longitudinal fissures, being almost without transverse ones, and the *Loxa* bark of a brown color, externally ash-gray, with numerous, remote, transverse fissures, should have the preference, and be employed. The inferior barks should be rejected; such as are very smooth, or scaly wrinkled, externally, and have a liver color, and such in which the resinous circle is wanting in the middle layer, and the outer surface is of a dark color.

---

* Cinchona pallida, U. S. Pharmacopœia.

Cortex Chinæ ruber.

[Red Cinchona]. Rothe Chinarinde.

Cinchona succirubra *Pavon*, **and of other imperfectly described species.**

In flat, or somewhat curved or arched pieces of bark, from a half to two centimetres thick. The outer layer is of a dark brownish-red color, covered with oval, warty protuberances, frequently furrowed longitudinally, being either of a corky or compact consistence. The liber is thick, brownish-red, and fibrous, having a splintery fracture, and, on a transverse section, the bast-cells are arranged radially in the parenchyma.

The taste is astringent and very bitter, when the bark is chewed. Thin, quilled, light and pale pieces are to be rejected.

The bark should not be confounded with *Cinchona rubiginosa*, which is more fibrous and of almost an orange-red color.

Cortex Cinnamomi Cassiæ.

[Cassia Bark]. Zimmtkassie.

[*Chinese Cinnamon*]. *Chinesischer Zimmt. Cortex Cinnamomi Chinensis.*

Cinnamomum Cassia *Blume.*

The inner bark of the branches, about one and a half millimetres thick, in single rolled quills, and of a yellowish-brown color. The fibres, on the outer surface, are pale, scattered, and rather indistinct. The fracture is nearly smooth, the odor agreeable, and when the bark is chewed its taste is burning, astringent, non-mucilaginous, and sweetish.

Cortex Cinnamomi Zeylanici.

[Ceylon Cinnamon]. Zeylonzimmt.

Cinnamomum acutum. Cortex Cinnamomi acuti.

Cinnamomum Zeylanicum *Breyn;* (**Laurus Cinnamomum** *Linn*).

The inner bark of the younger branches, consisting of very thin, brittle quills, several being rolled together; having a pale yellowish-brown color, and exhibiting on the outer surface conspicuous, scattered, pale fibres. It has a closely fibrous fracture, a strong, peculiar, fragrant odor, and sweet taste; producing a burning sensation when chewed, being only slightly astringent.

Cortex Frangulæ.

[EUROPEAN BUCKTHORN]. Faulbaumrinde.

[*European Black Alder*]. *Cortex Rhamni Frangulæ.*

Rhamnus Frangula *Linn.*

A quilled bark, about one millimetre in thickness, gray or brownish-gray externally, with small, white, warty protuberances, which are generally lengthened transversely. The old bark is slightly fissured, covered with a very thin corky layer, which is separable in scales, and of a purplish color on the inside. The bark is internally brownish-yellow; it has a smooth, reddish-brown inner surface, and a fibrous fracture; the fibres are of a lemon-yellow color.

The bark of the younger trunks, and the larger branches of the indigenous shrub, are gathered in the spring.

Cortex Fructus Aurantii.

[BITTER ORANGE PEEL]. Pomeranzenschale.

Cortex Pomorum Aurantii.

Citrus vulgaris *Risso.* *a.* **amara** *Linn.*

The peel of the ripe fruit, in elliptical sections, each cut consisting of the fourth part of the rind; when dry it is yellowish-brown, glandular; spongy and white internally, of a bitter taste, and grateful odor.

Only the peel, freed from the interior skin, the *Flavedo* [yellow part of the rind], should be used; but the *Flavedo* of the thin, hard, Curaçao orange peel, with a dirty-green color externally, should not be substituted, neither the rind of the [sweet] orange from *Citrus Aurantium* Risso, which is distinguished by its orange-yellow color, and also by its odor.

Cortex Fructus Citri.

[LEMON PEEL]. Citronenschale.

Citrus Limonum *DC.* **et Citrus medica** *Linn.*

The dried rind of the ripe fruit, occurring in commerce in spiral pieces; externally glandular and of a lemon-yellow color; having a thin spongy, white interior layer. It has a grateful odor and a weak, bitter taste.

Cortex Fructus Juglandis.

[GREEN WALNUT HULLS]. Grüne Wallnussschale.

Cortex Nucum Juglandis.

Juglans regia *Linn.*

The exterior green pericarp (hull) of the ripe drupe (stone-fruit). It separates easily from the bony nut-shell; is fleshy, green on the outside, whitish and somewhat spongy internally, and tinges the skin brown. It has an aromatic odor, and a somewhat astringent, bitter and weak acidulous taste.

Cortex Mezerei.

[MEZEREON BARK]. Seidelbastrinde.

Kellerhalsrinde.

Daphne Mezereum *Linn.*

A bark consisting of thin, rather long strips, having a brownish periderm, which can be readily removed, and underneath a thinner green layer. The liber is very tough, flexible, finely fibrous, yellowish-white, and of a silky lustre. Its taste is very acrid.

The bark should be gathered in the early spring, from the trunk and larger branches.

The bark of *Daphne Laureola* Linn., may also be used; it is distinguished from the former by its green liber.

Cortex Quercus.

[OAK BARK]. Eichenrinde.

Quercus pedunculata *Ehrhart,* **and Quercus sessiliflora** *Martyn.*

A bark from one to two millimetres in thickness, the outer portion is brittle, the inner tough and band-like fibrous, having a very thin, separable, shining, silver-gray periderm, a brown middle layer, and a brownish or yellowish liber, narrowly tesselated on the transverse section; it separates later in thin, narrow, flexible bands. The taste is astringent and bitter when chewed.

The bark is gathered in the spring from young trunks, and from not too old branches, of trees growing abundantly in Germany.

Cortex Radicis Granati.

[BARK OF POMEGRANATE ROOT]. Granatwurzelrinde.

Punica Granatum ***Linn.***

In longitudinally curved or quilled pieces of bark, of different sizes, rarely more than one and a half millimetres in thickness; on the outer surface they are ruggedly-warty, more or less fissured, grayish or brownish-yellow; internally greenish-yellow and not striated radially. The inner surface is of a pale cinnamon color, smooth or covered with very thin, yellowish-white adhering splinters. The bark has a uniform fracture, and an astringent and mildly bitter taste when chewed.

Crocus.

[SAFFRON]. Safran.

Crocus Sativus ***Linn.***

The dried stigmas about three centimetres long, almost tubular, but are compressed into a somewhat semi-cylindrical form; they widen towards their upper extremity, are finely notched, have a deep orange-yellow color and generally remain attached to the very short, yellow style. Saffron has a fragrant odor and a somewhat bitter taste, and when chewed colors the saliva a reddish-yellow.

It should be protected from the light, and care should be taken against adulterations.

Cubebæ.

[CUBEBS]. Cubeben.

Baccæ v. Fructus Cubebæ.

Cubeba officinalis ***Miquel.*** **(Piper Cubeba** ***Linn. fil.*****)**

The dried, somewhat hard drupes, covered with a thin, pericarp, nearly globular, rugous-reticulated, one-seeded and attenuated at the base into a stipe four or six millimetres long; of a dark, grayish-brown color, and of about the size of black pepper; burning when chewed, and of a strong aromatic odor.

Cuprum aceticum.

[ACETATE OF COPPER]. Krystallisirter Grünspan.

[*Neutral Acetate of Copper. Crystallized Verdigris*]. *Ærugo crystallisata.*

In dark-green, prismatic crystals, efflorescent in the air, having a nauseous metallic taste; soluble in fourteen parts of cold water, in five parts of boiling water, and also in alcohol to which has been added a small quantity of acetic acid. Acetate of copper is wholly soluble in water of ammonia, with an intense blue color. An aqueous solution, heated with an excess of caustic soda, and filtered, should not become turbid with hydrosulphuric acid.

It should be *cautiously* preserved in well-closed vessels.

Cuprum aluminatum.

Lapis divinus.

Take of Pure Sulphate of Copper, ... 16
Nitrate of Potassium, ... 16
Alum, each, *sixteen parts.* 16

Powder, and mix the ingredients, then fuse them in a porcelain capsule at a gentle heat. Remove them from the fire and add rapidly a mixture of

Camphor, powdered, ... 1
Alum, powdered, each, *one part.* 1

Pour the mass into a porcelain vessel, and when cold, break it into pieces.

It forms a light-blue mass, having the odor of camphor; soluble in sixteen parts of water, leaving but a slight residue.

It should be *cautiously* preserved in well-closed vessels.

Cuprum oxydatum.

[BLACK OXIDE OF COPPER]. Kupferoxyd.

A black powder, which should not contain particles soluble in water. It is completely soluble in diluted sulphuric acid.

When concentrated sulphuric acid is poured upon it, no nitrous vapors should be developed. When dissolved in diluted sulphuric acid, decomposed with a large excess of hydrosulphuric acid, the filtrate leaves no residue after evaporation.

It should be *cautiously* preserved.

Cuprum sulfuricum ammoniatum.

[AMMONIO-SULPHATE OF COPPER]. Schwefelsaures Kupferoxyd-Ammoniak.

Ammoniacum cuprico-sulphuricum. Cuprum ammoniacale.

Take of Pure Sulphate of Copper *one part*. . . . 1
Dissolve it, by stirring, in
Water of Ammonia *three parts*. . . . 3
To the filtered liquid add of
Alcohol *six parts*. 6

Collect the resulting precipitate on a filter, and dry it between bibulous paper without heat.

A dark-blue, crystalline powder, efflorescent in the air, soluble in one and a half parts of cold water, which solution has an alkaline reaction, is clear, but upon the addition of a greater portion of water becomes turbid.

It should be *cautiously* preserved in well-closed vessels.

Cuprum sulfuricum crudum.

[CRUDE SULPHATE OF COPPER]. Roher Kupfervitriol.

[Blue Vitriol]. Blauer Vitriol. Vitriolum Cupri.

In blue, rhomboidal-prismatic crystals, or in crystalline, translucent masses; soluble in four parts of cold, and in two parts of boiling water.

It is almost entirely soluble in water of ammonia with a dark-blue color.

It should be *cautiously* preserved.

Cuprum sulfuricum purum.

[PURE SULPHATE OF COPPER]. Reiner Kupfervitriol.

In translucent, rhomboidal crystals, of a rich deep-blue color; they effloresce slowly in dry air; are soluble in three and a half parts of cold water, and in equal parts of hot water; insoluble in alcohol.

The aqueous solution, to which has been added a large excess of water of ammonia, is of a dark-blue color. The watery solution, on being first acidulated with a little sulphuric acid, and then decomposed with an excess of hydrosulphuric acid, yields a filtrate, which leaves no residue on evaporation.

It should be *cautiously* preserved.

Decocta.

[DECOCTIONS]. Abkochungen.

Decoctions, that are ordered without a given quantity of the substance to be used, are made, so, that from *one part* of the substance *ten parts* of colature (strained decoction) are gained. To prepare *ten parts* of colature of a *concentrated decoction, one and a half parts* of the substance are used; and to prepare *ten parts* of colature of a *highly concentrated decoction, two parts* of the substance must be taken.

The quantity of medicinally *active* substances must always be prescribed by the physician.

The substance, from which the decoction is to be made, is put in a suitable vessel and cold water poured upon it, the vessel is kept in a steam-bath for half an hour, stirring occasionally, and the liquid is then, while still warm, strained by expression.

For the preparation of Decoction of Salep, see Mucilage of Salep.

Decoctum Sarsaparillæ compositum fortius.

[ZITTMANN'S STRONGER DECOCTION]. Stärkeres Zittmann'sches Decoct.

Take of Sarsaparilla Root, cut, *one hundred parts*. . . 100
Pour upon it
Common Water *two thousand and six hundred parts*, ... 2600
digest for twenty-four hours, then add of
Sugar, powdered, ... 6
Alum, powdered, each, *six parts*, . . . 6
and heat them in a covered vessel, in a steam-bath, for three hours, stirring frequently. Towards the end of the boiling, add of
Anise, bruised, ... 4
Fennel Seed, bruised, each, *four parts*, . . . 4
Senna, cut, *twenty-four parts*, ... 24
Liquorice Root, cut, *twelve parts*. 12

Strain by expression, and set aside for a short time. The clear, decanted liquid should be *two thousand and five hundred parts*. 2500

When not otherwise directed, a colature of *two thousand and five hundred grammes* is divided. into *eight portions.*

N.B.—When *Decoctum Zittmanni* is prescribed, it is prepared in a similar manner, except to the sugar and alum is added of

Mild Chloride of Mercury *four parts*, . . 4
Cinnabar (Red Sulphide of Mercury) *one part*, 1

inclosed in a linen bag.

Decoctum Sarsaparillæ compositum mitius.

[ZITTMANN'S MILDER DECOCTION]. Milderes Zittmann'sches Decoct.

Take the residue of the Stronger Decoction, and
Sarsaparilla Root, cut, *fifty parts*. . . . 50

Pour upon them
Common Water *two thousand and six hundred parts*, ... 2600

and expose to the heat of a steam-bath, for three hours, in a covered vessel, stirring frequently. Toward the end of the operation, add of

Lemon Peel, ... 3
Cassia Bark, ... 3
Small Cardamoms, ... 3
Liquorice Root, each, cut and bruised, *three parts*. 3

Strain by expression, and set aside for a short time. The clear decanted liquid should be *two thousand and five hundred parts*. 2500

When not otherwise directed, a colature of *two thousand and five hundred grammes*, is divided into *eight portions*.

Dextrinum.

[DEXTRIN]. Dextrin.

Take of Potato Starch *one hundred and fifty parts*, . 150
Cold Distilled Water *seven hundred and fifty parts*, ... 750
Crystallized Oxalic Acid *four parts*. . . . 4

Mix carefully, and expose them, in a covered vessel, to the heat of a steam-bath, stirring frequently, so long as unaltered starch can be detected by solution of iodine. Then add of

Precipitated Carbonate of Lime,

a quantity sufficient to neutralize the acid, and set aside for two days in a cool place. Then filter the liquid and evaporate it, by means of a steam-bath, until a mass is formed which no longer adheres to the fingers. It is then drawn out into threads, and dried at a gentle heat.

Dextrin should be dry, inodorous, easily powdered, similar to gum arabic, and wholly soluble in an equal weight of water, which solution, on the addition of a double quantity of alcohol, throws down a copious precipitate. An aqueous solution is not colored blue by tincture ef iodine.

It should be preserved in well-closed vessels.

Elæosacchara.

[OLEOSACCHARATES]. Oelzucker.

Take of Best White Sugar, powdered, *two grammes*, . 2
Any of the essential oils *one drop*.

Mix them.

Electuarium e Senna.

[CONFECTION OF SENNA]. Sennalatwerge.

Electuarium lenitivum.

Take of Senna, powdered, *ten parts*, ... 10
Coriander Seed, powdered, *one part*. . . 1
Mix and add of
Simple Syrup *fifty parts*, ... 50
Purified Tamarind Pulp *fifteen parts*. . . 15

Prepare a confection by means of a steam-bath. It is greenish-brown and should be preserved in a dry and cool place.

Electuarium Theriaca.

[THERIACK]. Theriak.

Theriaca. Electuarium theriacale.

Take of Opium, powdered, *one part*, ... 1
Sherry Wine *three parts*. 3
Macerate for a day, stirring occasionally, then add of
Angelica Root, powdered, *six parts*, . . . 6
Virginia Snake Root, powdered, *four parts*, . 4
Valerian Root, powdered, ... 2
Squill, powdered, ... 2
Zedoary Root, powdered, ... 2
Cassia Bark, powdered, each, *two parts*, . . 2
Small Cardamoms, powdered, ... 1
Myrrh, powdered, ... 1
Pure Protosulphate of Iron, powdered, each, *one part*, ... 1
Purified Honey *seventy-two parts*. 72

Make into a confection, which should be preserved in a cool place. It has a brown color.

One hundred parts contain one part of opium.

Elemi.

[ELEMI]. Elemi.

Gummi v. Resina Elemi.

From an undetermined Plant growing in Yucatan.

In irregular, solid, or, occasionally, soft, slightly translucent masses, of a greenish-yellow or orange-yellow color, and strong, peculiar odor. It melts readily, and is soluble in boiling alcohol.

Other species of Elemi, and masses mixed with pieces of bark, should be rejected.

Elixir amarum.

[BITTER ELIXIR]. Bitteres Elixir.

Take of Extract of Buck-bean, ... 2
Extract of Orange Peel, each, *two parts*. . . 2
Dissolve them in
Peppermint Water, ... 16
Diluted Alcohol, each, *sixteen parts*, . . . 16
and add of
Spirit of Ether (*Spiritus æthereus*) *one part*. . 1

Bitter Elixir has a dark-brown color.

Elixir Aurantii compositum.

[HOFFMANN'S STOMACH ELIXIR]. Hoffmann'sches Magenelixir.

Elixir viscerale Hoffmanni.

Take of Orange Peel *six parts*,	6
Cassia Bark, bruised, *two parts*,	2
Pure Carbonate of Potassium *one part*,	1
Sherry Wine *fifty parts*.	50

Macerate for eight days, express and strain.

To the colature add of

Extract of Gentian,	1
Extract of Wormwood,	1
Extract of Buck-bean,	1
Extract of Cascarilla, each, *one part*.	1

After repose, filter.

It forms a clear liquid, of a brown color, having a peculiar, aromatic odor, and a bitter taste.

It should be preserved in a well-closed vessel.

Elixir Proprietatis Paracelsi.

[ACIDULATED ELIXIR OF ALOES]. Saures Aloëelixir.

Take of Aloes, coarsely powdered,	2
Myrrh, coarsely powdered, each, *two parts*,	2
Saffron, powdered, *one part*.	1

Pour upon them

Alcohol *twenty-four parts*,	24
Diluted Sulphuric Acid *two parts*.	2

Macerate for eight days and filter.

It forms a clear reddish-brown liquid.

Elixir e Succo Liquiritiæ.

[PECTORAL ELIXIR]. Brustelixir.

Elixir e Succo Glycyrrhizæ.

Elixir pectorale.

Take of Purified Liquorice *two parts*.	2

Dissolve it in

Fennel Water *six parts*,	6

add of

Anisated Spirits of Ammonia *two parts*.	2

It forms a cloudy, brown liquid, which must be shaken up before dispensing.

It should be preserved in well-closed vessels.

Emplastrum ad Fonticulos.

[FONTANEL PLASTER. ISSUE PLASTER]. Fontanellpflaster.

Take of Burgundy Pitch *three parts*, ... 3
Suet *one part*, ... 1
Lead Plaster *thirty-six parts*. 36

Melt them at a moderate heat, and spread the mass, in uniform thickness, on thin linen cloth; double the spread cloth a number of times, and, having placed wax-paper between each layer, perforate it with a cylindrical iron punch, three centimetres in diameter.

They form very adhesive circular pieces of plaster.

Emplastrum adhæsivum.

[ADHESIVE PLASTER]. Heftpflaster.

Take of Crude Oleic Acid *eighteen parts*, ... 18
add, while stirring constantly, of
Litharge, in very fine powder, *ten parts*. . . 10

Heat them by means of a steam-bath, until a plaster is formed. Before cooling, add of
Resin *three parts*, ... 3
Suet *one part*. 1

A yellowish and very adhesive plaster.

Emplastrum adhæsivum Edinburgense.

[EDINBURGH ADHESIVE PLASTER]. Edinburger Heftpflaster.

It is prepared like Adhesive Plaster, but in place of Resin and Suet, take
Black Pitch, *three parts*. 3

A dark-brown and very adhesive plaster.

Emplastrum adhæsivum Anglicum.

[English Court Plaster]. Englisches Pflaster.

Taffetas adhæsivum.

Take of Isinglass *ten parts*. 10

Dissolve it in a sufficient quantity of

Common Hot Water,

so that a colature [solution] is obtained, which should be

one hundred and twenty parts. 120

Take *sixty parts* of this solution, and by means of a brush, spread a sufficient number of coatings on stretched silk (taffeta), which should measure, for each *thirty grammes* of Isinglass, one hundred and four (104) centimetres in length and forty-two (42) centimetres in breadth.

Each coating should be allowed to dry.

The remaining *sixty parts* of this Isinglass solution are gradually mixed with

Alcohol *forty parts* 40

Glycerin *one part*, ... 1

and this mixture is brushed over the fabric in the same manner [as the previous solution.]

Finally, the reverse side of the fabric is coated with *a sufficient quantity* of Tincture of Benzoin, and the plaster is then well dried, and preserved in a dry place.

It is lustrous, and, when moistened, becomes very adhesive to the skin.

Emplastrum Ammoniaci.

[Ammoniac Plaster]. Ammoniakpflaster.

Take of Yellow Wax, ... 4

Burgundy Pitch, each, *four parts*. 4

Melt, strain through a linen cloth, and to the partially-cooled mass add of

Purified Ammoniac *six parts*, ... 6

Purified Galbanum *two parts*, ... 2

previously dissolved by means of a steam-bath, in

Turpentine *four parts*. 4

The plaster is formed into rolls.

It has a greenish color.

Emplastrum aromaticum.

[AROMATIC PLASTER]. Aromatisches Pflaster.

[*Stomach Plaster*]. *Magenpflaster*. *Emplastrum stomachicum*.

Take of Yellow Wax *thirty-two parts*,	32
Suet *twenty-four parts*,	24
Turpentine *eight parts*.	8
Melt them, and to the partially-cooled mass, add of	
Oil of Nutmeg (expressed) *six parts*,	6
Olibanum, powdered, *sixteen parts*,	16
Benzoin, powdered, *eight parts*,	8
Oil of Peppermint,	1
Oil of Cloves, each, *one part*.	1

They are intimately mixed, formed into rolls, and kept in wax-paper.

Aromatic Plaster is grayish-brown and has an aromatic odor.

Emplastrum Belladonnæ.

[BELLADONNA PLASTER]. Belladonnapflaster.

Take of Yellow Wax *four parts*,	4
Turpentine,	1
Olive Oil, each, *one part*.	1

Melt them, and to the partially cooled mass add gradually of

Belladonna Leaves, powdered, *two parts*.	2

It forms a brownish-green plaster.

It should be preserved in a dry place.

Emplastrum Cantharidum ordinarium.

[CANTHARIDES PLASTER]. Spanischfliegenpflaster.

[*Blistering Plaster*]. *Blasenpflaster*. *Emplastrum vesicatorium ordinarium*.

Take of Cantharides, coarsely powdered, *two parts*,	2
Common Olive Oil *one part*.	1

Mix, and place them in a steam-bath for several hours, then add of

Yellow Wax *four parts*,	4
Turpentine *one part*,	1

melt and mix well together. When cold, form the plaster into rolls.

The plaster is greasy and soft to the touch, interspersed, regularly, with shining green particles.

It should be preserved in a dry place.

Emplastrum Cantharidum perpetuum.

[PERPETUAL CANTHARIDES PLASTER]. Immerwährendes Spanischfliegenpflaster.

Take of Resin, ...	50
Yellow Wax, each, *fifty parts*, ...	50
Turpentine *thirty-seven parts*, ...	37
Burgundy Pitch *twenty-five parts*, . . .	25
Suet *twenty parts*.	20
Melt them with a gentle heat, and add of	
Cantharides, in very fine powder, *eighteen parts*,	18
Euphorbium, in very fine powder, *six parts*. .	6

It forms a greenish-black plaster.

Emplastrum Cerussæ.

[WHITE LEAD PLASTER]. Bleiweisspflaster.

Froschlaichpflaster. Emplastrum album coctum.

Take of Litharge, in very fine powder, *ten parts*, . .	10
Olive Oil *twenty-five parts*.	25

Boil them in a copper vessel, stirring constantly, until the Litharge is dissolved, adding from time to time a little warm water, then add of

White Lead, in very fine powder, *eighteen parts*, 18

and continue the boiling, and the adding of a moderate quantity of warm water, to prevent burning, until a plaster is formed, which, when cold, is formed into rolls.

The plaster is white, heavy, hard, and, when moderately heated, tenacious.

Emplastrum Conii.

[CONIUM PLASTER]. Schierlingspflaster.

Emplastrum Cicutæ.

It is prepared from Powdered Conium Leaves, like Belladonna Plaster.

Emplastrum Conii ammoniacatum.

[CONIUM PLASTER WITH AMMONIAC]. Mit Ammoniakgummi versetztes Schierlingspflaster.

Emplastrum Cicutæ cum Ammoniaco.

Take of Ammoniac, powdered, ... 2
Vinegar of Squill, each, *two parts*. . . . 2

Evaporate by a gentle heat to a somewhat tough consistence, then mix them intimately with

Conium Plaster *nine parts*. 9

It is formed into rolls.

The plaster is somewhat soft, not very tenacious, and has a dirty-green fracture.

Emplastrum fœtidum.

[ASSAFETIDA PLASTER]. Stinkasantpflaster.

Emplastrum Asæ fœtidæ.

Take of Yellow Wax, ... 4
Burgundy Pitch, each, *four parts*. . . . 4

Melt, strain, and to the partially cooled mass add of

Assafetida, powdered, *six parts*, . . . 6
Ammoniac, powdered, *two parts*, . . . 2

previously dissolved, by means of a steam-bath, in

Turpentine *four parts*. 4

It forms a tenacious, yellowish plaster.

Emplastrum fuscum.

[BREAST PLASTER]. Schwarzes Mutterpflaster.

Emplastrum Matris fuscum Ph. Saxon.

Take of Red Oxide of Lead, in very fine powder, *thirty-two parts*, ... 32
Olive Oil *sixty-four parts*. 64

Boil them in a copper kettle, stirring constantly, until the mass assumes a dark-brown color.

Then add of

Yellow Wax *sixteen parts*. 16

Pour it into paper capsules.

A dark-brown, soft, and tenacious plaster.

Emplastrum fuscum camphoratum.

[UNIVERSAL PLASTER]. Universalpflaster.

Schwarzes Mutterpflaster. Nürnberger Pflaster. Emplastrum nigrum s. universale s. Noricum. Emplastrum fuscum Ph. Bor. Emplastrum Minii adustum.

Take of Emplastrum fuscum *one hundred parts*. . . . 100
Melt, and add of
Camphor *one part*, ... 1
previously dissolved in a small quantity of Olive Oil, then pour the plaster into paper capsules.

It must have the odor of camphor.

Emplastrum Galbani crocatum.

[GALBANUM PLASTER WITH SAFFRON]. Mit Safran versetztes Mutterharzpflaster.

Emplastrum de Galbano crocatum.

Take of Lead Plaster *twenty-four parts*, ... 24
Yellow Wax *eight parts*. 8
Melt them, and to the partially cooled mass add of
Purified Galbanum *twenty-four parts*, . . 24
previously dissolved, by means of a steam-bath, in
Turpentine *six parts*, ... 6
then add of
Saffron, powdered, *one part*, ... 1
which has been rubbed into a pulp with a small quantity of Alcohol.

It is formed into rolls.

The plaster is yellowish-brown, and softens readily.

Emplastrum Hydrargyri.

[MERCURIAL PLASTER]. Quecksilberpflaster.

Emplastrum mercuriale.

Take of Mercury *eight parts*, ... 8
Turpentine *four parts*. 4

The mercury is intimately rubbed together with the turpentine, to which has been added a little Oil of Turpentine, and then to the mass is added, gradually, under constant stirring, of
Lead Plaster *twenty-four parts*, ... 24
Yellow Wax *six parts*, ... 6
which have been previously melted together.

The plaster, after cooling, is formed into rolls.

It has a gray color, and no globules of mercury should be detected by the naked eye.

Emplastrum Hyoscyami.

[Hyoscyamus Plaster]. Bilsenkrautpflaster.

It is prepared from Powdered Hyoscyamus Leaves, like Belladonna Plaster.

Emplastrum Lithargyri compositum.

[Compound Diachylon Plaster]. Gummipflaster.

[***Compound Lead Plaster***]. ***Zugpflaster. Emplastrum Plumbi compositum. Emplastrum diachylon compositum.***

Take of Lead Plaster *twenty-four parts*, ... 24
Yellow Wax *three parts*. 3

Melt them together with a moderate heat, and to the partially cooled mass add of

Ammoniac, powdered, ... 2
Galbanum, powdered, ... 2
Turpentine, each, *two parts*, ... 2

which have been previously melted in a steam-bath.

Mix them well, and form the plaster into rolls after cooling.
It forms a brownish-yellow, tenacious plaster.

Emplastrum Lithargyri molle.

[White Breast Plaster]. Weisses Mutterpflaster.

Emplastrum Matris album Ph. Saxon.

Take of Lead Plaster *three parts*, ... 3
Lard *two parts*, ... 2
Suet, ... 1
Yellow Wax, each, *one part*. 1

Melt them together, strain, and pour into paper capsules.
A somewhat yellowish plaster.

Emplastrum Lithargyri simplex.

[LEAD PLASTER]. Bleipflaster.

Emplastrum Plumbi simplex. Emplastrum diachylon simplex.

Take of Olive Oil,
Lard,
Litharge, in very fine powder, each, *equal parts.*

Boil them with a moderate heat, stirring constantly with a spatula, and adding occasionally a little warm water until a plaster is formed, which make into rolls.

Lead Plaster is white and tenacious; it is not greasy, and contains no undissolved oxide of lead.

Emplastrum Meliloti.

[MELILOT PLASTER]. Melilotenpflaster.

It is prepared from powdered Melilot, like Belladonna Plaster.

Emplastrum Mezerei cantharidatum.

[CANTHARIDATED PLASTER OF MEZEREON]. Mit Canthariden versetztes Seidelbastpflaster.

Take of Cantharides, coarsely powdered, *thirty grammes,*	30
Mezereon Bark, cut and bruised, *ten grammes,* .	10
Acetic Ether *one hundred grammes,* . . .	100

Macerate for eight days, shaking frequently; then express, and dissolve in the filtered liquid,

Sandarac *four grammes,*	4
Elemi, ...	2
Resin, each, *two grammes.*	2

Spread this solution, by means of a brush, on stretched silk (taffeta), measuring three thousand square centimetres; the silk having been previously covered with a solution of

Isinglass *twenty grammes,*	20
Distilled Water *two hundred grammes,* . .	200
Alcohol *fifty grammes.*	50

Emplastrum Minii rubrum.

[RED-LEAD PLASTER]. Rothes Mennigepflaster.

Emplastrum s. Ceratum de Minio rubrum.

Take of Yellow Wax, ... 100
Suet, each, *one hundred parts*, ... 100
Provence Olive Oil *forty parts*. 40

Melt them together, and to the partially cooled mass, add of

Red-Lead, in very fine powder, *one hundred parts*, ... 100
Camphor *three parts*. 3

which were previously rubbed together, and thoroughly mixed with

Provence Olive Oil *sixty parts*. 60

It forms a uniform mass, which pour into paper capsules. The Plaster has a red color and the odor of camphor.

Emplastrum opiatum.

[OPIUM PLASTER]. Opiumpflaster.

Hauptpflaster. Emplastrum Cephalicum.

Take of Elemi *eight parts*, ... 8
Turpentine *fifteen parts*, ... 15
Yellow Wax *five parts*. 5

Melt them together with a moderate heat, and, to the strained mass, add of

Olibanum, powdered, *eight parts*, ... 8
Benzoin, powdered, *four parts*, ... 4
Opium, powdered, *two parts*, ... 2
Balsam of Peru *one part*, ... 1

and make into a plaster.

Opium Plaster is brown and tenacious.

Emplastrum oxycroceum.

[Saffron Plaster. Oxycroceum Plaster]. Safranpflaster.

Oxycroceumpflaster. Emplastrum Galbani rubrum.

Take of Yellow Wax, ... 6
Resin, ... 6
Burgundy Pitch, each, *six parts*. . . . 6

Melt them together with a moderate heat, and, to the strained mass, add of

Ammoniac, powdered, ... 2
Galbanum, each, *two parts*, ... 2

previously dissolved in

Turpentine *three parts*. 3

Then add of

Mastic, powdered, ... 2
Myrrh, powdered, ... 2
Olibanum, powdered, each, *two parts*, . . 2
Saffron, powdered, *one part*, ... 1

previously rubbed together.

The Plaster is formed into rolls.

It is reddish-brown and tenacious.

Emplastrum Picis irritans.

[Irritant Pitch Plaster]. Reizendes Pechpflaster.

Take of Burgundy Pitch *thirty-two parts*, . . . 32
Yellow Wax, ... 12
Turpentine, each, *twelve parts*. 12

Melt them together by means of a water-bath, and add of

Euphorbium, in very fine powder, *three parts*. . 3

The Plaster has a yellow color.

Emplastrum saponatum.

[Soap Plaster]. Seifenpflaster.

Take of Lead Plaster *seventy-two parts*, ... 72
Yellow Wax *twelve parts*. 12

Melt them with a moderate heat, and to the partially cooled mass, add, while stirring, of

Castile Soap, well dried and powdered, *six parts*, 6
Camphor *one part*, ... 1

which has been previously dissolved in a little Olive Oil. The plaster is formed into rolls after cooling.

Soap Plaster is whitish, somewhat soft, and not slippery.

Emulsiones.

[EMULSIONS]. Emulsionen.

Emulsions of Seeds are made, when not otherwise directed, by using *one part* of Seeds, ... 1
and Water sufficient, that *ten parts* 10
of *colature* (strained emulsion) are procured.

Oil-Emulsions are made, when not expressly otherwise directed, by using of

Any desired oil *two parts*, ... 2
Gum Arabic, powdered, *one part*, ... 1
Distilled Water *seventeen parts*. . . . 17

Remark.—When no other oil is prescribed, for an Oil-Emulsion, Almond Oil is invariably used.

Emulsio Amygdalarum composita.

[COMPOUND ALMOND EMULSION]. Zusammengesetzte Mandelemulsion.

Take of Sweet Almonds *four parts*, ... 4
Hyoscyamus Seed *one part*, ... 1
Diluted Bitter Almond Water *sixty-four parts*, 64
make an emulsion, and add of
Best White Sugar *six parts*, ... 6
Calcined Magnesia *one part*. 1

The emulsion is prepared only when wanted for dispensing.

Euphorbium.

[EUPHORBIUM]. Euphorbium.

[***Gum Euphorbium***].

Euphorbia resinifera ***Berg.***

In dirty-yellowish, round, somewhat three-cornered pieces, from the size of a lentil to that of a hazelnut, frequently perforated with from one to three holes; friable, translucent, and inodorous. Its powder produces very violent sneezing. It is partially soluble in water, alcohol, and in ether.

It should be separated from the admixture of small branches and fruit, as much as possible, and *cautiously* preserved.

Extracta.

[EXTRACTS]. Extrakte.

The substances used for the preparation of Extracts should be finely and uniformly cut or bruised; and when distilled water is not directed to be used, a water, as free as possible from carbonate of lime, should be taken.

Maceration should be conducted at a temperature of between 10° and 20° C.; digestion at a heat of from 35° to 40° C. Frequent stirring, or shaking, must be used in both cases.

The aqueous liquids are evaporated immediately to one-third their volume, and are then set aside, in a cool place, for several days and decanted from their sediment. The alcoholic and ethereal liquids are decanted, filtered, and then, by means of a steam-bath, brought to the consistence of an extract, while stirring constantly. The alcohol and ether, used, may be previously distilled off.

The steam-bath should be so arranged, that the temperature of the liquids, to be evaporated, does not exceed the boiling point of water. In evaporating ethereal liquids, the temperature must not exceed 50° C.

Extracts are prepared of three degrees of consistence:

1. *Thin extracts*—of the consistence of fresh honey.
2. *Thick extracts*—which, when cold, cannot be poured from a vessel, but may still be drawn out in threads by means of a spatula.
3. *Dry extracts*—which are pulverizable. They are prepared by evaporation in a porcelain vessel, and brought to the consistence of a tough mass, which becomes friable when cold. The mass is removed with a spatula, while still warm, drawn into thin ribbons and dried on paper with a moderato heat, reduced to a coarse powder, and immediately inclosed in a vessel, previously warmed.

The thick extracts are preserved in tightly-covered, glazed earthen or porcelain vessels. The thin and dry extracts are kept in cork-stoppered, glass vessels; all must be kept in a cool and dry place.

The extracts should possess the taste and odor of the substances from which they were prepared, and be free from copper and tin.

It is recommended that a small quantity of the *thick* narcotic extracts be mixed with Dextrin, and kept ready prepared, as follows: *Ten parts* of powdered Dextrin are gradually mixed with an equal quantity of extract, in a warm, porcelain capsule, the mass is then dried at a temperature of 40° to 50° C., and the heat continued, until there is no longer a diminution of weight.

The dried and still warm mass is rubbed, and mixed with a sufficient quantity of powdered Dextrin, to make its weight double that of the extract employed.

Of this powder, double the weight of *thick* extract prescribed is dispensed.

Extractum Absinthii.

[EXTRACT OF WORMWOOD]. Wermuthextrakt.

Take of Wormwood *two parts*. 2
Pour upon it
Alcohol, ... 6
Common Water, each, *six parts*, . . . 6
digest for twenty-four hours, and express. Treat the residue in the same manner with
Alcohol, ... 3
Common Water, each, *three parts*. . . . 3

Evaporate the mixed and filtered liquids to the consistence of a *thick* extract.

Extract of Wormwood is greenish-brown, forming a turbid solution with water.

Extractum Aconiti.

[EXTRACT OF ACONITE]. Eisenhutextrakt.

Take of Aconite Root, coarsely powdered, *two parts*. . 2
Pour upon it
Diluted Alcohol *four parts*, ... 4
macerate for eight days in a covered vessel, stirring frequently, and then express. Treat the residue in the same manner with
Diluted Alcohol *three parts*. 3

Evaporate the mixed and filtered tinctures, with a moderate heat, to the consistence of a *thick* extract.

Extract of Aconite is yellowish-brown, forming a yellowish-brown and turbid solution with water.

It should be *cautiously* preserved.

Extractum Aloes.

[EXTRACT OF ALOES]. Aloëextrakt.

Take of Aloes, powdered, *one part*. 1
Pour upon it
Distilled Water *four parts*. 4

Macerate for forty-eight hours, stirring frequently. Then set the mixture aside to settle, afterwards strain, and convert the clear liquid into a *dry* extract.

Extract of Aloes is in the form of a yellowish-brown powder, forming a turbid solution with water.

Extractum Aloes Acido sulfurico correctum.

[VITRIOLATED EXTRACT OF ALOES]. Mit Schwefelsäure versetztes Aloëextrakt.

Take of Extract of Aloes *eight parts*. 8
Pour upon it
Distilled Water *thirty-two parts*, ... 32
add, drop by drop, of
Pure Sulphuric Acid *one part*, ... 1
then evaporate the liquid, in a porcelain vessel, to a *dry* extract.

The extract is in the form of a dark-brown powder, forming a somewhat cloudy solution with water.

Extractum Aurantii Corticis.

[EXTRACT OF ORANGE PEEL]. Pomeranzenschalenextrakt.

Take of Orange Peel *one part*. 1
Pour upon it
Alcohol, ... 2
Common Water, each, *two parts*, ... 2
digest for three days, then express.
Pour upon the residue
Alcohol, ... 1
Common Water, each, *one part*. 1

Digest again for three days, and express.

From the mixed and filtered liquids, prepare a *thick* extract.

Extract of Orange Peel is reddish-brown, forming a nearly clear solution with water.

Extractum Belladonnæ.

[EXTRACT OF BELLADONNA]. Tollkirschenextrakt.

Take of Belladonna Leaves and Branches of the fresh, flowering plant *twenty parts*. . . . 20
Sprinkle with
Common Water *one part*, ... 1
bruise them in a stone mortar and express forcibly.
Pour upon the residue
Common Water *three parts*, ... 3
and repeat the process. Heat the mixed liquids to 80° C., strain and evaporate, by means of a steam-bath, to *two parts*, ... 2
then add of
Alcohol *two parts*, ... 2
mix, set aside for twenty-four hours, stirring occasionally, and strain through a linen cloth.
Rub the residue with
Diluted Alcohol *one part*, ... 1
and again express. Mix the liquids, filter, and evaporate to the consistence of a *thick* extract.

Extract of Belladonna is dark-brown, forming a brown and almost clear solution with water.

It should be *cautiously* preserved.

Extractum Calami.

[EXTRACT OF CALAMUS]. Kalmusextrakt.

It is prepared from Calamus Root, like Extract of Wormwood.

It is reddish-brown, forming a turbid solution with water.

Extractum Cannabis Indicæ.

[EXTRACT OF INDIAN HEMP]. Indischer Hanfextrakt.

Take of Indian Hemp *one part*. 1
Pour upon it
Alcohol *six parts*, ... 6
digest for three days, and express.
Pour upon the residue
Alcohol *four parts*, ... 4
digest as before, and express. From the mixed and filtered tinctures prepare a *thick* extract.

Extract of Indian Hemp is dark-brown, and insoluble in water.

It should be *cautiously* preserved.

Extractum Cardui benedicti.

[EXTRACT OF BLESSED THISTLE]. Kardobenediktenextrakt.

Take of Blessed Thistle *one part*. 1
Pour upon it
Hot Water *six parts*, ... 6
digest for six hours, and express. Pour upon the residue
Hot Water *three parts*, ... 3
again digest as before, and express.

From the mixed liquids prepare a *thick* extract.

The Extract is brown, forming a turbid solution with water.

Extractum Carnis Liebig.

[EXTRACT OF MEAT]. Fleischextrakt.

Extractum Carnis.

A brown extract-like mass, having the agreeable odor of roasted meat, forming readily a clear solution with water. The aqueous solution, with the addition of a little common salt, has the flavor of beef-broth. One hundred parts of the extract should not lose, at the temperature of 110° C., more than twenty-two parts of moisture, and, after combustion, there should be left not less than eighteen parts of ashes, which contain but a small quantity of chloride of sodium. One hundred parts of the extract, digested in alcohol, should yield a liquid which, on being filtered and evaporated, should leave an extract amounting to no less than fifty-six parts.

Extractum Cascarillæ.

[EXTRACT OF CASCARILLA]. Kaskarillextrakt.

Take of Cascarilla Bark, coarsely powdered, *one part*. . 1
Pour upon it
Boiling Water *four parts*, ... 4
set them aside for twenty-four hours, then express.
Pour upon the residue
Boiling Water *two parts*, ... 2
digest, and again express. Allow the mixed liquids to settle, and evaporate the clear portion to the consistence of a *thick* extract.

Extract of Cascarilla is dark-brown, forming a turbid solution with water.

Extractum Centaurii.

[Extract of European Centaury]. Tausendgüldenkrautextrakt.

It is prepared from European Centaury, like Extract of Blessed Thistle.

The Extract is reddish-brown, forming a turbid solution with water.

Extractum Chamomillæ.

[Extract of Chamomile]. Kamillenextrakt.

Take of German Chamomile *two parts*. 2

Pour upon it

Alcohol, ... 8

Common Water, each, *eight parts*, ... 8

digest for twenty-four hours, then express.

Pour upon the residue

Alcohol, ... 4

Common Water, each, *four parts*, ... 4

again digest for twenty-four hours, and express.

From the mixed liquids prepare a *thick* extract.

The Extract is greenish-brown, forming a turbid solution with water.

Extractum Chelidonii.

[Extract of Celandine]. Schöllkrautextrakt.

It is prepared from the flowering Celandine, like Extract of Belladonna.

It is dark-brown, forming a turbid solution with water.

Extractum Chinæ fuscæ.

[EXTRACT OF CINCHONA]. Chinaextrakt.

Take of Brown [Pale, U. S. P.] Cinchona *one part.* . 1
Pour upon it
Diluted Alcohol *four parts,* 4
digest for twenty-four hours, stirring occasionally, and express. Pour upon the residue
Diluted Alcohol *two parts,* 2
again digest for twenty-four hours, and express.

From the mixed and filtered liquids prepare a *thick* extract.

The Extract is brown, forming a turbid solution with water.

Extractum Chinæ frigide paratum.

[COLD-PREPARED EXTRACT OF CINCHONA]. Kaltbereitetes Chinaextrakt.

Take of Brown [Pale, U. S. P.] Cinchona *two parts.* . 2
Pour upon it
Distilled Water *twelve parts,* 12
macerate for two days, and express. Macerate the residue in a similar manner with
Distilled Water *six parts,* 6
and express forcibly. Mix, and allow the liquid to settle, pour off the clear portion, and evaporate to one and a half parts, which strain, after cooling, and evaporate to the consistence of a *thick* extract.

The Extract is reddish-brown, forming a turbid solution with water.

Extractum Cinæ.

[EXTRACT OF SANTONICA]. Zittwerblüthenextrakt.

Take of Santonica (*Flores Cinæ*) *two parts.* 2
Pour upon it
Ether, ... 3
Alcohol, each, *three parts,* 3
macerate for three days, pour off the liquid, express the residue, and repeat the process with
Ether, ... 2
Alcohol, each, *two parts.* 2

From the mixed and filtered tinctures prepare a *thin* extract.

Extract of Santonica is dark-brown, and insoluble in water.

Extractum Colocynthidis.

[Extract of Colocynth]. Koloquintenextrakt.

Take of Colocynth, freed from seed, and coarsely cut,
two parts. 2

Pour upon it
Diluted Alcohol *twelve parts*, ... 12

digest for several days in a moderately warm place, stirring occasionally, and then express forcibly. Pour upon the residue
Diluted Alcohol, ... 5
Common Water, each, *five parts*. 5

Digest for twenty-four hours, stirring frequently, and express.

Mix the liquids, allow them to settle, decant the clear portion from the sediment, strain, and make a *dry* extract.

A yellowish-brown powder, forming a turbid solution with water.

It should be *cautiously* preserved.

Extractum Colocynthidis compositum.

[Compound Extract of Colocynth]. Zusammengesetztes Koloquintenextrakt.

Take of Extract of Colocynth *three parts*, ... 3
Aloes, powdered, *ten parts*, ... 10
Extract of Rhubarb *five parts*, ... 5
Resin of Scammony *eight parts*. 8

Sprinkle them with diluted alcohol, mix, and dry the mixture with a gentle heat.

It forms a coarse, brown powder.

Preserve it *cautiously*.

Extractum Colombo.

[Extract of Columbo]. Kolomboextrakt.

It is prepared from Colombo Root, like Extract of Orange Peel, excepting that it is evaporated to a *dry* extract.

A yellowish-brown powder, forming a turbid solution with water.

Extractum Conii.

[EXTRACT OF CONIUM]. Schierlingsextrakt.

It is prepared from fresh Conium leaves, like Extract of Belladonna.

It is brown, forming an almost clear solution with water.

It should be *cautiously* preserved.

Extractum Cubebarum.

[EXTRACT OF CUBEBS]. Kubebenextrakt.

It is prepared from Cubebs, like Extract of Santonica.

It is brown and insoluble in water.

Extractum Digitalis.

[EXTRACT OF DIGITALIS]. Fingerhutextrakt.

It is prepared from the fresh leaves and branches of the flowering Digitalis, like Extract of Belladonna.

It is brown, forming a turbid solution with water.

It should be *cautiously* preserved.

Extractum Dulcamaræ.

[EXTRACT OF BITTERSWEET]. Bittersüssextrakt.

It is prepared from the twigs of Bittersweet, like Extract of Blessed Thistle, except *four parts* of Hot Water are used in the first digestion and *two parts* in the second.

The Extract is reddish-brown, forming a turbid solution with water.

Extractum Fabæ Calabaricæ.

[EXTRACT OF CALABAR BEAN]. Kalabarbohnenextrakt.

Extractum Physostigmatis.

Take of Calabar Bean, coarsely powdered, *one part*. . 1
Pour upon it
Diluted Alcohol *five parts*, ... 5
digest for twenty-four hours, and strain with expression.
Pour upon the residue
Diluted Alcohol *three parts*, ... 3
and operate as before. Reduce the mixed and filtered liquids to the consistence of a *thick* extract, by means of a steam-bath, while stirring constantly.

It should be *cautiously* preserved.

Extractum Ferri pomatum.

[FERRATED EXTRACT OF APPLES]. Aepfelsaures Eisenextrakt.

Take of Sour Apples *fifty parts*. 50

Convert them into a soft pulp, which mix with cut straw and express. Set the liquid aside to settle, decant from the sediment, filter and heat it by means of a steam-bath, with the addition of
Powdered Iron *one part*, ... 1
or as much as will be acted upon, leaving a small portion undissolved. To the solution, when cold, add a quantity of Water sufficient to make the liquid amount to *forty-eight parts*, then filter and reduce to the consistence of a *thick* extract.

The Extract has a greenish-black color, forming a nearly clear solution with water.

It contains from *seven* to *eight per cent.* of iron, and sometimes much less, according to the acidity of the apples employed, and the amount of acid developed by fermentation.

Extractum Filicis.

[EXTRACT OF MALE FERN]. Wurmfarnextrakt.

Take of Male Fern Root, recently dried and powdered, *one part.* 1

Pour upon it

Ether *three parts,* 3

and macerate for three days. Decant the liquid, express the residue, and pour upon it

Ether *two parts.* 2

After due maceration, express again, and from the clear, decanted and mixed tinctures, prepare a *thin* extract.

Extract of Male Fern is greenish, and insoluble in water.

Extractum Gentianæ.

[EXTRACT OF GENTIAN]. Enzianextrakt.

Take of Gentian Root *one part.* 1

Pour upon it

Common Cold Water *six parts,* . . . 6

macerate for forty-eight hours, and then express.

Pour upon the residue

Common Cold Water *three parts,* . . . 3

macerate for twelve hours, and again express.

From the mixed and strained liquids prepare a *thick* extract.

Extract of Gentian is brown, forming a clear solution with water.

Extractum Graminis.

[EXTRACT OF COUCH-GRASS]. Queckenextrakt.

Take of the Root of Couch-Grass, finely cut, *one part,* . 1

Common Hot Water *six parts.* 6

Digest for six hours and strain. Evaporate the colature immediately to the consistence of syrup. Mix *one part* of this extract with *four parts* of Cold Distilled Water; filter and evaporate to the consistence of a *thick* extract.

The Extract is reddish-brown, forming a clear solution with water.

Extractum Gratiolæ.

[EXTRACT OF HEDGE-HYSSOP]. Gottesgnadenkrautextrakt.

It is prepared from fresh Hedge-Hyssop, like Extract of Belladonna.

The Extract is brown, forming a brown, turbid solution with water.

It must be *cautiously* preserved.

Extractum Helenii.

[EXTRACT OF ELECAMPANE]. Alantwurzelextrakt.

It is prepared from Elecampane Root, like Extract of Orange Peel.

The Extract is brown, forming a turbid solution with water.

Extractum Hyoscyami.

[EXTRACT OF HYOSCYAMUS]. Bilsenkrautextrakt.

It is prepared from the fresh leaves and small branches of the flowering Hyoscyamus, like Extract of Belladonna.

The Extract is of a greenish-brown color, forming a brown and turbid solution with water.

It should be *cautiously* preserved.

Extractum Lactucæ virosæ.

[EXTRACT OF ACRID LETTUCE]. Giftlattichextrakt.

It is prepared from the fresh flowering Acrid Lettuce, like Extract of Belladonna.

The Extract is brown, forming a nearly clear solution with water.

It should be *cautiously* preserved.

Extractum Ligni Campechiani.

[EXTRACT OF LOGWOOD]. Campecheholzextrakt.

Take of Logwood, chipped, *one part*, ... 1
Common Water *eight parts*. 8
Boil to one-half, strain, and boil the wood again with
Common Water *six parts*. 6

From the mixed and decanted clear liquids, prepare a *dry* extract.

A reddish-brown powder, forming a turbid solution with water.

Extractum Liquiritiæ Radicis.

[EXTRACT OF LIQUORICE ROOT]. Süssholzextrakt.

Extractum Glycyrrhizæ.

It is prepared from Liquorice Root, like Extract of Gentian.

The Extract is yellowish-brown, forming a clear solution with water.

Extractum Malti.

[EXTRACT OF MALT]. Malzextrakt.

Take of Barley Malt, bruised, ... 1
Common Water, each, *one part*. 1
Mix, set aside for three hours, then add of
Common Water *four parts*, ... 4
digest for an hour, at a temperature not exceeding 65° C.; then heat the mass to the boiling point, and strain immediately by expression.

Evaporate the clear liquid as rapidly as possible, stirring constantly, to the consistence of a *thick* extract.

Extract of Malt is yellowish-brown, having an agreeable, sweet taste.

It should be preserved in a cool place.

Extractum Malti ferratum.

[FERRATED EXTRACT OF MALT]. Eisenhaltiges Malzextrakt.

Take of Extract of Malt *ninety-five parts*, ... 95
mix it with
Pyrophosphate of Iron with Citrate of Ammonium *two parts*, ... 2
previously dissolved in
Distilled Water *three parts*. 3

The Extract has a sweetish, slightly ferruginous taste.

Extractum Mezerei.

[EXTRACT OF MEZEREON]. Seidelbastextrakt.

Take of Mezereon, finely cut, *one part*. 1
Pour upon it
Alcohol *four parts*, ... 4
digest for several days, stirring occasionally, then express strongly. Pour upon the residue
Alcohol *three parts*, ... 3
and manipulate as before.

Evaporate the mixed and filtered liquids to the consistence of a *thin* extract.

The Extract is of a greenish color, insoluble in water. It should be *cautiously* preserved.

Extractum Millefolii.

[EXTRACT OF YARROW]. Schafgarbenextrakt.

It is prepared from *equal portions* of the Flowers and the Leaves of Yarrow, like Extract of Wormwood.

The Extract is greenish-brown, forming a turbid solution with water.

Extractum Myrrhæ.

[EXTRACT OF MYRRH]. Myrrhenextrakt.

Take of Myrrh, bruised, *one part*. 1
Pour upon it
Distilled Water *five parts*, ... 5
and macerate for two days, stirring frequently. Prepare from the decanted and filtered liquid a *dry* extract.

In the form of a brownish-yellow powder with a reddish tint, forming a turbid solution with water.

Extractum Opii.

[EXTRACT OF OPIUM]. Opiumextrakt.

Take of Opium, powdered, *four parts*. 4
Pour upon it
Distilled Water *sixteen parts*, ... 16
macerate for twenty-four hours, stirring frequently, then strain with expression. Pour upon the residue
Distilled Water *twelve parts*, ... 12
again macerate for twenty-four hours and strain as before. Set aside the mixed liquids, that they may settle; filter, and convert them into a *dry* extract.

Extract of Opium is in the form of a reddish-brown powder, forming a turbid solution with water.

It should be *cautiously* preserved.

Extractum Pulsatillæ.

[EXTRACT OF PULSATILLA]. Küchenschellenextrakt.

It is prepared from the flowering Pulsatilla,* like Extract of Belladonna.

The Extract is brown, forming a turbid solution with water.

It should be *cautiously* preserved.

---

* *Vide* Herba Pulsatillæ.

Extractum Quassiæ.

[EXTRACT OF QUASSIA]. Quassiaextrakt.

It is prepared from Quassia Wood, like Extract of Logwood, except that it is brought to the consistence of a *thick* extract.

The Extract has a brown color, frequently interspersed with small crystals, forming a brown and turbid solution with water.

Extractum Ratanhæ.

[EXTRACT OF RHATANY]. Ratanhaextrakt.

Take of Rhatany Root, coarsely powdered, *one part*. . 1

Pour upon it

Common Water *four parts*. 4

Set aside for twenty-four hours, stirring frequently, and strain by expression. Pour upon the residue

Common Water *three parts*. 3

Set aside again for twenty-four hours and strain as before. Allow the mixed liquids to settle, pour off the clear portion, and convert it into a *dry* extract, by evaporating it in a porcelain capsule.

A shining, reddish-brown powder, forming a turbid solution with water.

Extractum Rhei.

[EXTRACT OF RHUBARB]. Rhabarberextrakt.

It is prepared from Rhubarb, like Extract of Wormwood.

The Extract is yellowish-brown, forming a turbid solution with water.

Extractum Rhei compositum.

[COMPOUND EXTRACT OF RHUBARB]. Zusammengesetztes Rhabarberextrakt.

Extractum catholicum s. panchymagogum.

Take of Extract of Rhubarb *three parts*, ... 3
Extract of Aloes *one part*. 1
Pour upon them
Distilled Water *four parts*, ... 4
allow them to soften in a moderately warm place, then add of
Jalap Soap *one part*, ... 1
previously dissolved in
Diluted Alcohol *four parts*. 4

Evaporate the mixture to the consistence of a *dry* extract.

A dark-brown powder, forming a brownish-yellow and turbid solution with water.

Extractum Sabinæ.

[EXTRACT OF SAVINE]. Sadebaumextrakt.

It is prepared from Savine, like Extract of Wormwood.

It has a greenish-brown color, forming a turbid solution with water.

It should be *cautiously* preserved.

Extractum Scillæ.

[EXTRACT OF SQUILL]. Meerzwiebelextrakt.

Take of Squill, coarsely powdered, *one part*, ... 1
Diluted Alcohol *four parts*. 4

Macerate for four days, then strain and express. Decant the clear liquid, filter, and convert it into a *thick* extract.

It is yellowish-brown, forming a nearly clear solution with water.

Extractum Secalis cornuti.

[EXTRACT OF ERGOT]. Mutterkornextrakt.

Ergotinum. Extractum hæmostaticum.

Take of Ergot, coarsely powdered, *one part*, ... 1
Distilled Water *two parts*. 2

Macerate for six hours, strain and express. Pour upon the residue
Distilled Water *two parts*, ... 2
and operate as before. Evaporate the mixed and filtered liquids to the consistence of a thin syrup, and add of
Diluted Alcohol *one part*, ... 1
mix, and set aside for a day, stirring frequently, then filter, and evaporate to the consistence of a *thick* extract.

The Extract has a reddish-brown color, forming a clear solution with water.

Extractum Senegæ.

[EXTRACT OF SENEKA]. Senegaextrakt.

It is prepared from Seneka Root, like Extract of Columbo.

A yellowish-brown powder, forming a turbid solution with water.

Extractum Stramonii.

[EXTRACT OF STRAMONIUM]. Stechapfelkrautextrakt.

It is prepared from the fresh leaves of Stramonium, like Extract of Belladonna.

The Extract is dark-brown, forming a nearly clear solution with water.

It should be *cautiously* preserved.

Extractum Strychni aquosum.

[Aqueous Extract of Nux Vomica]. Wässriges Krähenaugenextrakt.

Extractum Nucum vomicarum aquosum.

Take of Nux Vomica, coarsely powdered, *one part*. . 1
Pour upon it
Boiling Common Water *four parts*, . . . 4
set aside for twenty-four hours, stirring frequently, and then express. Pour upon the residue
Boiling Common Water *three parts*, . . 3
and operate as before.

Allow the mixed liquids to settle, decant the clear portion, and convert it into a *dry* extract.

A yellowish-brown powder, forming a greenish-white and turbid solution with water.

It should be *cautiously* preserved.

Extractum Strychni spirituosum.

[Alcoholic Extract of Nux Vomica]. Weingeistiges Krähenaugenextrakt.

Extractum Nucum vomicarum spirituosum.

Take of Nux Vomica, coarsely powdered, *two parts*. . 2
Pour upon it
Diluted Alcohol *four parts*, ... 4
digest for twenty-four hours, stirring occasionally; then pour off the clear liquid, and express. Pour again upon the residue
Diluted Alcohol *three parts*, ... 3
and operate as before.

Evaporate the mixed and filtered tinctures to a *dry* extract.

A brown powder, forming a turbid solution with water, having a very bitter taste.

It should be *cautiously* preserved.

Extractum Taraxaci.

[EXTRACT OF DANDELION]. Löwenzahnextrakt.

It is prepared from the dried entire flowering plant of Dandelion, like Extract of Blessed Thistle.

The Extract is brown, forming a nearly clear solution with water.

Extractum Trifolii fibrini.

[EXTRACT OF BUCKBEAN]. Fieberkleeextrakt.

It is prepared from Buckbean leaves, like Extract of Blessed Thistle.

The Extract is dark-brown, forming a clear solution with water.

Extractum Valerianæ.

[EXTRACT OF VALERIAN]. Baldrianextrakt.

It is prepared from Valerian Root. It is made into a *thick* extract, like Extract of Orange Peel.

The Extract is dark-brown, forming a turbid solution with water.

Faba Calabarica.

[CALABAR BEAN]. Kalabarbohne.

Semen Physostigmatis.

Physostigma venenosum ***Balfour.***

The seeds are oval or oblong, more or less kidney-shaped, somewhat compressed; about four centimetres in length, two centimetres in breadth, and eleven millimetres in thickness; covered with a brown, slightly shining, granular, wrinkled integument (testa), inclosing two, oval, whitish, brittle cotyledons. The seeds are convex on the one side, and more or less sinuous on the other, exhibiting a deeply furrowed margin of the hilum.

The seeds should be *cautiously* preserved.

Farina Hordei præparata.

[PREPARED BARLEY FLOUR]. Präparirtes Gerstenmehl.

Barley Flour is introduced into a cylindrical, tinned vessel, and pressed, so as to have two-thirds of the vessel filled. The closed vessel is then exposed to the heat of a steam-bath for thirty hours. When cold, the upper layer is removed and rejected, and the remaining reddish-yellow mass is converted into a powder, and preserved in a dry place.

Fel Tauri depuratum siccum.

[REFINED DRY OX-GALL]. Trockne gereinigte Ochsengalle.

[***Purified Ox Bile***].

Take of Fresh Ox-gall,
Alcohol, each, *equal parts.*

Mix thoroughly, set aside a short time, then filter, and distill off the alcohol by means of a steam-bath.

Add gradually to the residue, stirring repeatedly, a sufficient quantity of moist animal charcoal, previously purified by hydrochloric acid, until a small portion, taken out and filtered, shows only a slight yellow color. The whole is then filtered, and the liquid converted into a *dry* extract.

It forms a yellowish-white powder, giving a clear solution, of the same color, both with alcohol and water. The powder attracts moisture readily, and leaves, after combustion, only a very little white residue, which has an alkaline reaction.

One hundred parts of fresh ox-gall yield about seven parts of refined dry ox-gall.

It should be preserved in well-closed vessels.

Fel Tauri inspissatum.

[INSPISSATED OX-GALL]. Eingedickte Ochsengalle.

[***Inspissated Ox Bile***].

Ox-gall is heated and then strained through linen cloth, and evaporated by means of a steam-bath, in a porcelain vessel, without stirring, to the consistence of a *thick* extract.

It has a brownish-green color, forming a clear, greenish solution with water.

Ferrum carbonicum saccharatum.

[SACCHARATED CARBONATE OF IRON]. Zuckerhaltiges kohlensaures Eisen.

Take of Pure Protosulphate of Iron *five parts*. . . . 5
Dissolve it in
Hot Distilled Water *twenty parts*, ... 20
then pour it into a solution of
Bicarbonate of Sodium *four parts*, ... 4
Warm Water *fifty parts*, ... 50
contained in a sufficiently capacious glass flask, with a narrow neck. Fill the empty part of the flask with boiling water, and set the mixture aside for two hours. Draw off the supernatant liquid from the precipitate, by means of a syphon, and then fill the flask again with distilled water, and shake it; pour the clear liquid off again, and repeat the operation until the decanted liquid shows but a slight turbidity with chloride of barium. Then introduce the precipitated mass, free from water, into a porcelain capsule, containing
Sugar, powdered, *eight parts*, ... 8
and by means of a steam-bath evaporate to dryness, and reduce to powder.

It has a greenish-gray color, and at first a sweetish taste, afterwards slightly ferruginous. Hydrochloric acid dissolves it with copious evolution of carbonic acid gas. This solution should scarcely become turbid on the addition of chloride of barium. Saccharated Carbonate of Iron contains twenty per cent. of carbonate of iron.

A brown preparation, that effervesces but slightly with acids, should be rejected.

It should be preserved in well-closed vessels.

Ferrum chloratum.

[PROTOCHLORIDE OF IRON]. Eisenchlorür.

Ferrum muriaticum oxydulatum.

Take of Pure Hydrochloric Acid *five hundred and twenty parts*, ... 520
introduce it into a sufficiently capacious flask, and add, in successive small portions, of
Iron, in wire or filings, *one hundred and ten parts*. 110

When the evolution of gas has nearly ceased, place the flask in a steam-bath for several hours; then filter from the undissolved portion of iron, and immediately evaporate, with a rather strong heat, in a porcelain vessel, until a pellicle begins to form. Then add of

Pure Hydrochloric Acid *one part*, . . . 1

evaporate the whole, stirring constantly, to a stiff pasty mass, which, when removed from the fire, solidifies into a saline mass. Powder, and introduce it into rather small, previously warmed bottles, which must be tightly closed.

A light-greenish, saline powder, forming a clear solution with an equal weight of water when acidulated with a few drops of hydrochloric acid. This solution should not become turbid on the addition of three times its volume of alcohol, nor afford a precipitate with chloride of barium.

Ferrum citricum oxydatum.

[CITRATE OF IRON]. Citronensaures Eisenoxyd.

Take of Citric Acid *one part*. . . . . , . . . 1

Dissolve it in

Distilled Water *four parts*, ... 4

and mix gradually with

Hydrated Oxide of Iron,

recently precipitated, and still moist, *a sufficient quantity*, so that after a digestion at a gentle heat, for some time, with repeated stirring, a small portion remains undissolved. The filtered liquid is then evaporated, at a moderate heat, in a porcelain capsule, to the consistence of a syrup and spread upon plates of glass or porcelain, and allowed to dry.

The salt consists of, mostly thin, dry, amorphous, translucent scales, of a brownish-red color, having a mildly ferruginous taste. It is readily and wholly soluble in cold water, yielding a yellowish solution, which affords no precipitate on the addition of water of ammonia.

It should be preserved in well-closed vessels.

Ferrum citricum ammoniatum.

[Citrate of Iron and Ammonium]. Citronensaures Eisenoxyd-Ammonium.

Ferrum citricum cum Ammonio citrico. Ferro-Ammonium citricum.

Take of Citric Acid *two parts*. 2
Dissolve it in
Distilled water *eight parts*, ... 8
mix gradually with
Hydrated Oxide of Iron,
recently precipitated and still moist, *a sufficient quantity*, so that after a digestion for some time, at a gentle heat, with repeated stirring, a small portion (of the oxide) remains undissolved. Then filter the solution, add a little water through the filter to wash it, and dissolve in the filtered liquid
Citric Acid *one part*, ... 1
and add of
Water of Ammonia,
a sufficient quantity, so that the ammonia shall be in slight excess. Then evaporate the liquid in a porcelain capsule, with a moderate heat, to the consistence of syrup, and spread it on glass or porcelain plates, and allow it to dry.

In dry, amorphous scales which are mostly thin and translucent, having a reddish-brown color, and at first an acrid, saline taste, afterwards slightly ferruginous.

The aqueous solution yields no precipitate on addition of water of ammonia, but when heated with solution of caustic potassa, peroxide of iron is thrown down with evolution of ammonia.

Ferrum iodatum.

[Iodide of Iron]. Eisenjodür. Jodeisen.

Take of Powdered Iron *three parts*, ... 3
Distilled Water *eighteen parts*, ... 18
Iodine *eight parts*. 8

Introduce them into a glass flask, heat the mixture moderately until a greenish liquid is produced, then filter and add a little water through the filter to wash it.

Eight parts of iodine employed, correspond to *ten parts* of iodide of iron.

Iodide of iron should be prepared *extempore* after this formula, and added to the mixtures prescribed by the physician. If it is to be added to a pill-mass, the liquid is previously evaporated to a proper consistence with a gentle heat.

Ferrum iodatum saccharatum.

[SACCHARATED IODIDE OF IRON]. Zuckerhaltiges Jodeisen.

Take of Powdered Iron *three parts*, ... 3
Distilled Water *ten parts*, ... 10
Iodine *eight parts*. 8

Introduce them into a glass flask, set aside in a warm place, agitate frequently, until the red color of the liquid is changed to a greenish color.

Then filter into a porcelain capsule, containing
Sugar of Milk, powdered, *forty parts*, 40
add a little distilled water through the filter to wash it, mix well and evaporate to dryness, by means of a steam-bath, stirring constantly, until it is reduced to a dry state, and then rub the mass to powder.

A yellowish-white powder, soluble in seven parts of water, forming almost a clear solution. It contains *twenty per cent.* of iodide of iron. An aqueous solution, mixed first with starch and then cautiously with chlorine water, is colored a deep blue.

It should be *cautiously* preserved in rather small, well-closed vessels.

Ferrum lacticum.

[LACTATE OF IRON]. Milchsaures Eisenoxydul.

A crystalline powder, of a light greenish-yellow color, nearly inodorous, sparingly soluble in alcohol, soluble in forty-eight parts of water, forming a greenish-yellow solution, which is scarcely rendered turbid by acetate of lead. When heated with solution of caustic soda and filtered, the filtrate, to which has been added a little sulphate of copper, and gently heated, does not coagulate, nor is it rendered turbid with a red coloration.

Ferrum oxydatum fuscum.

[HYDRATED OXIDE OF IRON. HYDRATED PEROXIDE OF IRON].
Eisenoxydhydrat.

Ferrum oxydatum hydratum. Ferrum hydricum.

Take of Solution of Persulphate of Iron *forty parts*, . 40
Distilled Water *one hundred and sixty parts*. . 160
Mix, and add of
Water of Ammonia *thirty-two parts*, . . . 32
diluted with
Distilled Water *sixty-four parts*, . . . 64
or so much ammonia that it shall be in slight excess. Collect the resulting precipitate on a filter, wash it with water, express, and dry it at a gentle heat.

It forms a very fine powder, of a reddish-brown color, yielding, with hydrochloric acid, a clear saffron-colored liquid, which, when diluted with twenty parts of water, must show but a slight turbidity on the addition of chloride of barium.

It should be preserved in a well-closed vessel.

Ferrum oxydatum saccharatum solubile.

[SACCHARATED OXIDE OF IRON]. Eisenzucker.

Take of Solution of Sesquichloride of Iron, . . . 20
Simple Syrup, each, *twenty parts*. . . . 20
Mix, and while stirring, add slowly of
Solution of Caustic Soda *forty parts*, . . 40
and set aside for twenty-four hours. Then pour the clear liquid into
Hot Distilled Water *three hundred parts*, . . 300
stir, and allow it to settle. Decant the supernatant liquid, and again pour distilled water upon the precipitate, collect it on a filter, and wash it with distilled water so long as the water runs off colorless, and gives a rather strong alkaline reaction. Allow the precipitate to drain, to free it from most of the water, mix it in a porcelain capsule with
Best White Sugar, powdered, *ninety parts*, . 90
and evaporate to dryness, by means of a steam-bath, stirring constantly. Then mix with
Best White Sugar, powdered, *a quantity sufficient* that the whole shall be *one hundred parts*. 100

Reduce the mass to powder, and preserve it in a well-closed vessel.

It forms a reddish powder, of a sweet and mild ferruginous taste. It is wholly soluble in five parts of water, yielding a reddish-brown liquid, having a feeble alkaline reaction. It contains three per cent. of metallic iron.

Ferrum phosphoricum.

[PHOSPHATE OF IRON]. Phosphorsaures Eisenoxydul.

Take of Pure Protosulphate of Iron *three parts*, . . 3
Dissolve it in
Distilled Water *eighteen parts*, ... 18
then add to the liquid a solution of
Phosphate of Sodium *four parts*, ... 4
Distilled Water *sixteen parts*. 16

The resulting precipitate is immediately collected on a filter, washed with water, dried at a temperature not exceeding 25° C., and reduced to powder.

It forms a very fine powder, of a grayish-blue color, which, when heated, turns to a grayish-green. It is insoluble in water; but diluted hydrochloric acid, with a gentle heat, dissolves it, forming a golden-yellow solution.

It should be preserved in a well-closed vessel.

Ferrum pulveratum.

[POWDERED IRON]. Eisenpulver.

Limatura Martis præparata.

A very fine, gray, heavy powder, of a metallic lustre. On the addition of hydrochloric acid, only traces of hydrosulphuric acid gas should be developed, which may be detected by paper saturated with a solution of subacetate of lead. When the solution, made with hydrochloric acid, is completely oxidized by nitric acid, and an excess of water of ammonia added, and filtered, the filtrate should not be rendered turbid by hydrosulphate of ammonium.

Ferrum pyrophosphoricum cum Ammonio citrico.

[PYROPHOSPHATE OF IRON WITH CITRATE OF AMMONIUM].

Pyrophosphorsaures Eisenoxyd mit citronensaurem Ammonium.

Take of Pyrophosphate of Sodium *eighty-four parts.* . 84
Dissolve it in
Distilled Water *five hundred parts,* 500
pour this solution gradually into
Solution of Sesquichloride of Iron *eighty-four parts,* 84
previously diluted with
Distilled Water *eight hundred parts.* 800

Add the resulting precipitate, well washed with water and still moist, to a solution consisting of
Citric Acid *twenty-six parts,* 26
Distilled Water *fifty parts,* 50
then add of
Water of Ammonia *so much*
that the ammonia shall be in slight excess. When the solution is completed, evaporate the yellowish liquid, with a gentle heat, to the consistence of syrup, and spread it in thin layers, on flat plates and dry it properly.

In thin, greenish-yellow scales, of a mild ferruginous taste, readily and completely soluble in water. The solution is not precipitated by water of ammonia, but, when heated with solution of caustic potassa, it yields, with the evolution of ammonia, a yellowish-white precipitate.

Ferrum reductum.

[REDUCED IRON]. Reducirtes Eisen.

[*Iron reduced by Hydrogen*]. *Ferrum Hydrogenio reductum.*

A very fine, black, heavy powder, without lustre. It is converted into peroxide of iron by heating it in the air. It is wholly soluble in diluted hydrochloric acid, with the evolution of perfectly inodorous hydrogen gas, forming a bluish-green solution, which is but slightly reddened by sulphocyanide of potassium.

When digested with aqueous solution of bromine at a gentle heat, it must not leave more than one half of the iron undissolved, which, however, should be perfectly soluble in hydrochloric acid.

Ferrum sesquichloratum.

[SESQUICHLORIDE OF IRON]. Krystallisirtes Eisenchlorid.

[Perchloride of Iron]. Ferrum muriaticum oxydatum.

A yellow, crystalline mass, deliquescing slowly in the air, wholly soluble in water, alcohol, and ether, having but a feeble odor of hydrochloric acid ($Fe_2 Cl_6 + 12 H_2 O$).

A solution with fifty parts of water is colored brown by ferridcyanide of potassium, but no blue precipitate should be thrown down. When mixed with a solution of protosulphate of iron, no blue coloration is produced on the cautious addition of pure concentrated sulphuric acid.

It should be preserved in a well-closed, glass-stoppered bottle.

Ferrum sulfuricum crudum.

[CRUDE PROTOSULPHATE OF IRON]. Eisenvitriol.

[Copperas. Green Vitriol]. Grüner Vitriol. Ferrum sulphuricum venale. Vitriolum Martis.

In crystalline masses, or in transparent, rhomboidal, prismatic crystals, of a green color. It is sometimes contaminated with copper or other metals, and is, therefore, unfit for medicinal use.

Ferrum sulfuricum oxydatum ammoniatum.

[SULPHATE OF IRON AND AMMONIUM]. Schwefelsaures Eisenoxyd-Ammonium.

Ammoniakalischer Eisenalaun.

Take of Solution of Persulphate of Iron *three hundred parts*, ... 300
Sulphate of Ammonium *twenty-eight parts*, . 28
Distilled Water *one hundred parts*. . . . 100

Mix them in a porcelain capsule, and evaporate to crystallization.

The crystals are allowed to form by the gradual cooling of the liquid, and, having poured off the mother liquor, are quickly washed with a little water, and dried at a gentle heat.

In octahedral crystals, of a pale amethyst-violet color, soluble in four parts of cold water. The aqueous solution gives the reactions of sesquioxide of iron, ammonia, and sulphuric acid. When heated with an excess of solution of caustic potassa, it liberates ammonia, and throws down a precipitate of hydrated sesquioxide of iron. The liquid separated by filtration, acidulated with hydrochloric acid, and then treated with carbonate of ammonium in excess, must not yield a white precipitate of hydrate of alumina.

It should be preserved in well-closed vessels.

Ferrum sulfuricum purum.

[PURE PROTOSULPHATE OF IRON]. Reines schwefelsaures Eisenoxydul.

[Sulphate of Iron]. Reiner Eisenvitriol. Vitriolum Martis purum.

In translucent crystals, or in crystalline powder, of a light bluish-green color, soluble in less than two parts of cold, and in equal parts of boiling water; insoluble in alcohol; efflorescent in dry air.

The characteristic marks of its purity are similar to those of powdered iron.

It should be preserved in small, well-closed vessels.

Ferrum sulfuricum siccum.

[DRIED PROTOSULPHATE OF IRON]. Entwässertes schwefelsaures Eisenoxydul.

Take of Pure Protosulphate of Iron *a desired quantity*. Expose it to a heat of 100° C., in a porcelain capsule, until it is changed to a whitish mass, then reduce it to powder, and preserve it in a well-closed vessel.

A fine, greenish-white powder, slowly soluble in water, without a residue.

Flores Arnicæ.

[ARNICA FLOWERS]. Wohlverleihblüthen.

Arnikablüthen.

Arnica montana *Linn.*

The florets are of a pale orange-yellow color, provided with hairy, scabrous, fragile pappus. They are pubescent at the ovary and inside the tube; the ray-florets are pistillate (female), ligulate, and three-toothed, about four millimetres broad. The disk florets are perfect (hermaphrodite), tubular, with a five-toothed margin. Only the rayed flower-heads, deprived of the involucre, should be dispensed. The flowers have an acrid, but mildly bitter taste, causing sneezing when rubbed between the fingers.

They should not be confounded with other flowers of the Composite family, from which they are sufficiently distinguished by the above-given characteristic marks; and they should not have been attacked by the black larvæ of the arnica fly, *Trypeta Arnica.*

Flores Aurantii.

[ORANGE FLOWERS]. Pomeranzenblüthen.

Citrus Aurantium *Risso,* **and amara** *Linn.*

The recent flowers, of a very fragrant odor, with oblong, somewhat fleshy, very white petals; not having the roseate tint on the outside like those of *Citrus Limonum* Risso. The flowers have polyadelphous stamens, one-styled ovary, and a small, toothed calyx.

Flores Chamomillæ Romanæ.

[CHAMOMILE. ROMAN CHAMOMILE]. Römische Kamille.

Anthemis nobilis *Linn.*

Flower-heads radiate, becoming double by cultivation; involucre imbricate; receptacle convex, and furnished with obtuse, lacerated paleæ (chaff). The disk-florets are tubular, yellow, but mostly converted into larger, white, ligulate florets without pappus. The flowers have a strong, aromatic odor, and a bitter taste. They should not be confounded with the much smaller and double ones of Fever-few (*Pyrethrum Parthenium* Smith), and Sneezewort (*Achillea Ptarmica* Linn.)

Flores Chamomillæ vulgaris.

[GERMAN CHAMOMILE]. Kamille.

Gemeine Kamille.

Matricaria Chamomilla ***Linn.***

Flower-heads radiate, with an imbricated involucre, and a conical, naked receptacle; ligulate, white ray-florets, and tubular yellow disk-florets, without pappus.

The flowers have a strong, peculiar odor, and a bitter taste.

They should not be confounded with the flowers of *Pyrethrum inodorum* Smith, and *Anthemis Cotula* and *arvensis* Linn. The flowers of *Pyrethrum inodorum* and *Anthemis arvensis* are larger, and have convex, medullary receptacles, which, besides, are chaffy in *Anthemis*. In the fetid flowers of *Anthemis Cotula* the receptacle is medullary, and provided with bristly chaff.

Flores Cinæ.

[SANTONICA. LEVANT WORMSEED]. Wurmsamen.

Zittwersamen. Semen vel Anthodia Cinæ. Semen Santonici. Semen sanctum.

An undetermined species of Artemisia; tribe Seriphidiæ.

The unexpanded, smooth flower-heads, having an oblong, prismatic shape, a greenish, yellowish, or brownish color; about two millimetres long, inclosing a few florets. The involucre is imbricated, consisting of keeled scales, with membranous margins, dotted on the dorsal side with minute, golden-yellow glands. The outer scales are ovate, and smaller than the inner, oblong ones. Santonica possesses a peculiar, camphorous, but disagreeable odor and taste.

The so-called *Levant Wormseed* should only be used; the old and brown should be rejected.

The flowers known as *India Wormseed*, which are larger, and have often open flower-heads, and are somewhat hairy, covered with larger glands; and the more globular, grayish, downy, known as *Barbary Wormseed*, should be rejected.

Flores Kosso.

[Koosso]. Kosso.

[*Cusso*]. *Kusso. Kossoblüthen. Flores Brayeræ anthelminthicæ.*

Hagenia Abyssinica *Willdenow*, (**Brayera anthelminthica** *Kunth*).

Compressed, branching, hairy, bracteate panicles of crowded female flowers. They are perigynous, bibracteolate, often deflorated; the roundish bracts, and the four or five outer, oblong, membranous, and reticulated sepals, of a reddish or greenish color, and about one centimetre long, are inclosed in a short, top-shaped, hairy involucre. The flowers possess a bitter, nauseous taste.

They should be preserved in well-closed vessels, protected from the light, and, before dispensing, freed from the larger branches of the panicle.

Flores Lavandulæ.

[Lavender Flowers.] Lavendelblüthen.

Flores Lavendulæ.

Lavandula officinalis *Chaix*, (**Lavendula vera** *DC.*)

Flowers blue, with a violet-hairy, striated, five-toothed calyx, the upper tooth the largest; corolla bilabiate. They have a penetrating, aromatic odor.

The flowers must be gathered before they are quite open.

Flores Malvæ arboreæ.

[Hollyhock Flowers]. Stockrosen.

Flores Malvæ hortensis vel Alceæ.

Althæa rosea *Cavanilles.*

Flowers with a double, tomentose calyx, of which the outer one is often six-cleft, and the inner one five-cleft; the corolla is malvaceous, of a dark-brown color, often double, about five centimetres long, having monadelphous stamens. The flowers are mucilaginous, and mildly astringent.

The fully opened and perfect flowers must be gathered; the mouldy and worm-eaten should be rejected.

Flores Malvæ vulgaris.

[COMMON MALLOW FLOWERS]. Gemeine Malvenblüthen.

Flores Malvæ silvestris.

Malva silvestris *Linn.*

Flowers with a double calyx, of which the outer one is three-parted, and the inner five-cleft, and a very delicate, five-petalled corolla, nearly two centimetres long, of a roseate color, which changes to a lilac by drying; having monadelphous stamens. The flowers are mucilaginous.

Flores Millefolii.

[YARROW FLOWERS]. Schafgarbenblüthen.

Summitates Millefolii.

Achillea Millefolium *Linn.*

Flower-heads radiate, small, with a few florets; the heads disposed in a corymb; receptacle chaffy; involucre ovoid, imbricated with roundish, subtomentose scales, having scarious margins. The florets are white, or rose-colored, without pappus; rays mostly five, pistillate, and very broadly ligulate; disk-florets few, tubular, perfect. The flowers have a bitter taste, and aromatic odor.

Flores Primulæ.

[COWSLIP. PRIMROSE FLOWERS]. Schlüsselblumen.

Flores Primulæ veris.

Primula officinalis *Jacq.* (**Primula veris** *Sm.*)

The corolla is funnel-shaped, about two and a half centimetres long, of a lemon-yellow color, with a concave, five-lobed border, marked with five saffron-yellow spots in the throat. For use they are separated from the calyx. They have a feeble, honey-like odor, and sweetish taste.

They should be gathered in April and May. They must not be confounded with the flowers of *Primula elatior* Jacq. (Ox-lip Primrose), having a corolla with an entire border.

Flores Rhœados.

[RED POPPY]. Klatschrosen.

Papaver Rhœas *Linn.*

The petals of Red Poppy are roundish, very delicate, attenuated at the base, about five centimetres broad, of a dull-purple color when dry, having frequently a black claw. They are nearly inodorous, somewhat mucilaginous, with a slightly bitter taste.

Discolored, mouldy, and worm-eaten petals should be rejected.

Flores Rosæ.

[PALE ROSE]. Rose.

[*Hundred-leaved Rose*]. *Centifolienrose.*

Rosa centifolia *Linn.*

The recent petals, concave, of a pale red color, having a very agreeable odor; when dry they are paler, and less fragrant. In preserving them with salt, two parts of the petals and one part of common salt are strewn in alternate layers, in a suitable vessel; the layers pressed down and loaded with stones, and the vessel kept in a cool place.

Flores Sambuci.

[ELDER FLOWERS]. Fliederblumen.

Hollunderblüthen.

Sambucus nigra *Linn.*

Five-branched, many-flowered cymes; corolla epigynous, rotate, of a yellowish-white color, having a peculiar taste and odor.

Elder Flowers should be gathered in dry weather, and dark ones must be rejected.

Flores Tiliæ.

[LINDEN FLOWERS]. Lindenblüthen.

Tilia ulmifolia and Tilia platyphyllos ***Scopoli.***

Three to seven-flowered cymose peduncle, which is connate one-half its length, to a dry, leaf-like, linear-oblong, net-veined bract, of a greenish-yellow color. The flowers are yellowish-white, with five petals and five sepals, numerous hypogynous stamens. The ovary is nearly globular, tomentose.

Linden Flowers have a feeble odor when dry, and a sweetish taste.

They should be preserved in well-closed vessels, and kept no longer than a year.

Flores Verbasci.

[COMMON MULLEIN FLOWERS]. Wollblumen.

Königskerzenblumen.

Verbascum thapsiforme ***Schrader,*** **and other species of Verbascum.**

Corolla rather large, rotate, nearly regular, of a golden-yellow color (stamens five), three upper ones whitish-downy, and shorter than the two lower ones, which are smooth; anthers, long decurrent. The flowers have a faint odor, are mucilaginous when chewed, and of a sweetish taste.

They should be gathered in dry weather, separated from the calyx, and preserved in well-closed vessels, which are warmed before the introduction of the flowers.

Folia Althææ.

[MARSHMALLOW LEAVES]. Altheeblätter.

Eibischkraut. Herba Althææ.

Althæa officinalis ***Linn.***

The leaves are petiolate, sub-cordate, pointed, three or five-lobed, or entire, dentate, and covered on both sides with a soft down. They are mucilaginous when chewed.

Folia Aurantii.

[ORANGE LEAVES]. Pomeranzenblätter.

Citrus vulgaris ***Risso.***

The leaves are oblong, pointed and smooth, exhibiting pellucid dots. The jointed petiole is provided with rather broad wings (lateral appendages), and is obovate or obcordate in form. The leaves have a bitterish taste, and, when rubbed, exhale a fragrant odor.

They should be collected in summer, and not be confounded with the leaves of *Citrus Limonum* and *medica* Risso, in which the wings of the petiole are much smaller, or entirely wanting.

Folia Belladonnæ.

[BELLADONNA LEAVES]. Tollkirschenblätter.

Belladonnablätter. Herba Belladonnæ.

Atropa Belladonna ***Linn.***

The leaves are oval, narrowing toward the petiole, entire, pointed, of a dark-green color on their upper surface. The younger leaves are pubescent, the older only slightly so on the nerves. They have a faint, narcotic odor, and a weak, disagreeable, somewhat bitter taste.

The leaves should be gathered from the perennial plant (growing spontaneously in the mountains of Middle and Southern Europe), while blossoming in the summer months, and be quickly dried; they have a dark-green color. They should be preserved in well-closed vessels.

The powder should be prepared from the recently dried leaves, and kept in a well-closed vessel, in a dark place.

Preserve them *cautiously.*

Folia Digitalis.

[DIGITALIS, OR FOXGLOVE LEAVES]. Fingerhutkraut.

Herba Digitalis purpureæ.

Digitalis purpurea ***Linn.***

The leaves are oblong, narrowing towards the petiole, crenate, wrinkled, more or less tomentose, especially on their under surface; they have a bitter nauseous taste.

The leaves must be gathered from the flowering plant, growing spontaneously, and not from the cultivated one; and should be dried in the shade, *cautiously* preserved in a vessel, protected from the light, and renewed once a year.

Folia Farfaræ.

[COLTSFOOT]. Huflattigblätter.

Herba Farfaræ vel Tussilaginis.

Tussilago Farfara *Linn.*

The leaves are roundish-cordate, angular-sinuate, toothed, light-green above, and covered with a whitish down beneath; of a bitter and slightly astringent taste.

They should be gathered in May, and not be confounded with the younger leaves of *Petasites officinalis* Mœnch, which are kidney-heart-shaped, and grayish-woolly beneath; nor with the kidney-shaped leaves of *Petasites tomentosus* DC.

Folia Hyoscyami.

[HYOSCYAMUS LEAVES]. Bilsenkraut.

[Henbane Leaves]. Herba Hyoscyami.

Hyoscyamus niger *Linn.*

The leaves are hairy, oblong-ovate, sinuate-dentate. They have a nauseous, narcotic odor.

They should be gathered from the spontaneously-growing, flowering plant, and be *cautiously* preserved, but not kept longer than a year.

Folia Juglandis.

[EUROPEAN WALNUT LEAVES]. Wallnussblätter.

Juglans regia *Linn.*

The leaves are impari-pinnate, consisting generally of nine large, oblong-ovate leaflets, bearded beneath at the angles of the veins; the lateral leaflets are only jointed. They have a peculiar odor, and a somewhat bitter taste.

The leaves should be gathered in June, quickly dried, and carefully preserved. The dried leaves should have a green color.

Folia Laurocerasi.

[Cherry-Laurel Leaves]. Kirschlorbeerblätter.

Prunus Laurocerasus *Linn.*

The recent leaves; they have a short petiole, are oblong, eight to sixteen centimetres long, remotely serrate, coriaceous, smooth, veined, and provided with glands on their lower surface towards the angles of the veins. The odor of the rubbed leaves does not differ from that of bitter almonds. The taste is bitter and astringent.

They should be gathered in July and August.

Folia Malvæ.

[Common Mallow]. Malvenblätter.

Herba malvæ.

Malva vulgaris *Fries,* (**Malva rotundifolia** *Bauhin*), **Malva silvestris** *Linn.*

Leaves with long petioles, nearly kidney-shaped, or heart-shaped, roundish, loosely hairy, five or seven-lobed. The lobes are serrate, broadly obtuse, or extended. The leaves are mucilaginous when chewed.

Folia Melissæ.

[Balm, or Melissa Leaves]. Melissenblätter.

Herba Melissæ.

Melissa officinalis *Linn. α.* **citrata** *Bischoff.*

The leaves are petiolate, ovate, or nearly heart-shaped, crenate-serrate, of a green color, paler beneath; glandular, and slightly hairy on the nerves. They have an agreeable odor, and a mildly bitter taste. They should not be confounded with the leaves of *Nepeta Cataria* Linn. *β. citriodora*, which are grayish-woolly underneath.

Folia Menthæ crispæ.

[CURLED-MINT]. Krauseminzblätter.

Herba Menthæ crispæ.

Mentha crispa *Linn.*, **et Mentha crispata** *Schrader.*

Leaves subsessile, cordate or rounded-ovate, blistered-wrinkled, wavy, incised-toothed, obtuse or pointed, hairy or smooth, glandular.

The leaves have a burning taste, when chewed, and a peculiar odor. They should be gathered during the summer months.

Folia Menthæ piperitæ.

[PEPPERMINT]. Pfefferminze.

Herba Menthæ piperitæ.

Mentha piperita *Linn.*

Leaves with rather long petioles; oblong, pointed, sharply-toothed, subglabrous, glandular, of a fragrant odor and camphorous taste, followed by a sensation of coolness in the mouth.

The leaves should be collected in the summer months, and should not be confounded with the leaves of *Mentha viridis* Linn., which are sessile and less aromatic.

Folia Nicotianæ.

[TOBACCO LEAVES]. Tabaksblätter.

Herba Tabaci.

Nicotiana Tabacum *Linn.*

Leaves large, oblong-lanceolate, entire, pointed, narrowing towards the base, with glandular hairs on their surface; brown when dried. They are acrid, when chewed, and have a peculiar odor.

The leaves of Virginia tobacco, of one year's growth, should only be employed.

Folia Rosmarini.

[ROSEMARY LEAVES]. Rosmarinblätter.

Herba Rosmarini vel Roris marini.

Rosmarinus officinalis *Linn.*

Leaves rigid, linear, rugose, glandular, revolute at the edge, hoary beneath, with a prominent nerve, having a camphorous odor and taste.

The leaves of the plant growing spontaneously in Southern Europe should have the preference.

Folia Rutæ.

[RUE LEAVES]. Rautenblätter.

Herba Rutæ.

Ruta graveolens *Linn.*

Leaves petiolate, nearly tripinnately parted, thickish, grayish-green, glandular; terminal segments spatulate.

The fresh leaves have a strong odor, and a burning, somewhat bitter taste, which become milder in the dried leaves.

They should be gathered before the plant is in blossom.

Folia Salviæ.

[SAGE LEAVES]. Salbeiblätter.

Herba Salviæ.

Salvia officinalis *Linn.*

Leaves petiolate, oblong, wrinkled, crenulate, and thinly tomentose. They have an aromatic odor, and a bitter, astringent taste.

The leaves should be gathered before the plant begins to blossom.

Folia Sennæ.

[SENNA]. Sennesblätter.

[Alexandria or Tripoli Senna]. Alexandrische odor Tripolitanische Sennesblätter.

Cassia lenitiva *Bischoff* (**Senna acutifolia** *Batka*).

Leaflets subcoriaceous, oval or oblong, widest in the middle, oblique at their base, pointed, mucronulate, veined, more or less puberulent, and of a pale, grayish-green color. They have a peculiar odor, and a somewhat bitter, nauseous taste. The Alexandria or Tripoli Senna should only be used, and it is not necessary that it shall be entirely free from the leaves of *Solenostemma Arghel* Hayne, which are rigid, lanceolate, with an equal base, one-nerved, glaucous, and pubescent; but the senna should be as free as possible from pods and leaf-stalks. The following kinds should not be employed: the leaflets of *Cassia angustifolia* Vahl, which are oblong-lanceolate, acute, widest at their base; the wild (inferior), East India or Mecca senna; the cultivated Tinnevelly senna, with large, unbroken leaflets; nor the obovate leaflets of *Cassia obovata* Colladon, commonly called Aleppo or Italian senna.

Senna leaves, known as small senna (*Senna parvæ*), consisting of fragmentary leaves, should not be employed, on account of their frequent adulteration.

Folia Sennæ Spiritu extracta.

[SENNA EXHAUSTED BY ALCOHOL]. Mit Spiritus ausgezogene Sennesblätter.

Senna leaves are macerated with *four parts* of Alcohol for two days, then expressed and dried.

Folia Stramonii.

[STRAMONIUM LEAVES]. Stechapfelblätter.

Herba Stramonii.

Datura Stramonium *Linn.*

Leaves petiolate, ovate, acute, sinuate-dentate, dark-green above, paler beneath, and puberulent on the nerves; having a narcotic odor, and a bitter, nauseous taste.

The leaves should be gathered when the plant is in blossom, and be *cautiously* preserved, but not kept longer than a year.

Folia Toxicodendri.

[POISON OAK. POISON IVY]. Giftsumachblätter.

Herba Rhois Toxicodendri.

Rhus Toxicodendron *Michaux.*

Leaves long-petiolate, ternate, with membranous, acute leaflets, the middle one being petiolate and oval, and the two lateral sessile, ovate, with unequal sides. The fresh leaves abound with an acrid juice, which darkens when exposed to the air, and, when applied to the skin, produces inflammation and swelling; the leaves should therefore not be touched with the bare hands.

They should not be confounded with the leaves of *Ptelea trifoliata* Linn., which are similar in appearance, but have all the leaflets sessile.

The leaves must be gathered in June and July, and be *cautiously* preserved, but not kept longer than a year.

Folia Trifolii fibrini.

[BUCKBEAN LEAVES]. Fieberkleeblätter.

Bitterklee. Dreiblatt. Herba Trifolii fibrini.

Menyanthes trifoliata *Linn.*

Leaves petiolate, ternate, with subsessile, thickish, oval or oblong, obtuse, slightly repand-crenate, smooth, and light-green leaflets. They have a very bitter taste.

They should be gathered in May and June.

Folia Uvæ Ursi.

[UVA URSI]. Bärentraubenblätter.

[*Bearberry Leaves*]. *Folia Arctostaphyli. Herba Uvæ Ursi.*

Arctostaphylos Uva Ursi *Sprengel* (**Arbutus Uva Ursi** *Linn.*)

Leaves coriaceous, obovate, entire, smooth, shining, and net-veined on both sides. Their taste is somewhat bitter and astringent.

They should not be confounded with the leaves of Cowberry (*Vaccinum Vitis-Idæa* Linn.), with revolute margins, beneath dull, veined, and marked with brown dots.

The leaves should be gathered in summer.

Fructus Anisi stellati.

[STAR-ANISE]. Sternanis.

Semen Anisi stellati.

Illicium anisatum *Loureiro.*

Carpels drupaceous, about eight in number, disposed in a star-like form; they are boat-shaped, compressed, rather hard, externally grayish-brown and wrinkled; internally smooth; one-seeded, and dehiscent at the upper suture. The seeds are compressed, chestnut-brown and shining. Star-Anise has a slightly acrid and sweetish taste, and an aromatic odor.

It should be as free as possible from stalks. The unripe, small, and shriveled carpels, and the slightly odorous, should be rejected.

Fructus Anisi vulgaris.

[ANISE]. Anis.

[*Aniseed. Anise Fruit*]. *Gemeiner Anis. Semen Anisi vulgaris.*

Pimpinella Anisum *Linn.*

The fruit (schizocarp) is broadly ovate, slightly compressed at the sides, densely covered with short, downy hairs; of a grayish-green color. It is about two millimetres long, consisting commonly of the adherent mericarps, which have five ridges and numerous vittæ (oil-tubes). They have a sweetish, somewhat burning taste when chewed. Their odor is aromatic.

The fruit should be perfectly ripe, and as free as possible from stalks, particles of earth, and other impurities.

Fructus Aurantii immaturi.

[ORANGE BERRIES]. Unreife Pomeranzen.

Aurantia immatura.

Citrus vulgaris *Risso* (**Citrus Aurantium,** *a.* **amara** *Linn.*)

The unripe, dried berries; globose, glandular, many-celled, hard; about the size of a cherry, of a dark-green color, having an aromatic odor, and a bitter taste.

Fructus Cannabis.

[HEMP-SEED]. Hanfsamen.

Hanfkörner. Semen Cannabis.

Cannabis sativa *Linn.*

The nutlets are broadly ovate, somewhat compressed, submarginate, smooth, and of a greenish-gray color, containing a single, oleaginous seed.

The old and rancid seeds should be rejected.

Fructus Capsici.

[CAPSICUM]. Spanischer Pfeffer.

[*Cayenne Pepper*]. ***Piper Hispanicum.***

Capsicum annuum et longum *Fingerhut.*

A juiceless, conical berry, generally of a red color, shining, supported by a slightly flat calyx; hollow, incompletely two to three-celled, with a thin, leathery pericarp. The seeds are flat, yellowish, and attached to a thick sporophore (placenta). Capsicum, when chewed, produces an acrid, burning sensation in the mouth, and, on being powdered, violent sneezing.

Fructus Cardamomi minores.

[SMALL CARDAMOM]. Kleiner Kardamom.

[***Officinal, or Malabar Cardamom***]. ***Semen Cardamomi minoris. Cardamomum minus vel Malabaricum.***

Elettaria Cardamomum *White et Matoni.*

A chartaceous, triangular, striated, three-celled capsule, from eight to twelve millimetres long, of a straw color, containing small, hard, brown, wrinkled seeds, with obtuse angles, being furrowed on one side, and white internally. The seeds have a strong, aromatic odor, and a burning taste when chewed.

Capsules, deprived of their seeds, should not be bought; neither should the less aromatic, Ceylon, or Long cardamom, nor the round Java cardamom, be employed.

Only the seeds, separated from the capsules, must be used for the preparation of powder.

Fructus Carvi.

[CARAWAY SEEDS]. Kümmel.

*[Caraway Fruit]. **Kümmelsamen. Semen Carvi.***

Carum Carvi *Linn.*

The fruit is oblong, much compressed on the sides, about four millimetres long. The mericarps are readily separable; they are narrow, lessening towards both ends, with five whitish, filiform ridges, and broad, brownish channels; in each one a single vitta. They have a slightly burning taste when chewed, and a peculiar odor.

The fruit should be entirely ripe, and as free as possible from stalks and other impurities.

Fructus Ceratoniæ.

[ST. JOHN'S BREAD]. Johannisbrot.

[Sweet-pod]. Siliqua dulcis.

Ceratonia Siliqua *Linn.*

Legumes, with cross septa; very much compressed, juiceless, fleshy; externally of a chestnut-brown color, and obtusely four-cornered on a cross section. The mesocarp is somewhat thick, lacunose, of a brownish color, and sweet taste. The cells are one-seeded, and covered with a paper-like endocarp. The seeds are flattened, very hard, and shining.

Very dry and worm-eaten pods should be rejected.

Fructus Colocynthidis.

[COLOCYNTH]. Koloquinten.

Colocynthis. Poma Colocynthidis.

Citrullus Colocynthis *Arnott* (Cucumis Colocynthis *Linn.*)

The dried baccate fruit, deprived of the rind; it is globose, about the size of an apple, having a very light, spongy, whitish, and very bitter pulp, and numerous parietal seeds, nidulant in the pulp.

Very fleshy colocynth, with comparatively few seeds, is preferred; hard and brown should be rejected.

It should be *cautiously* preserved, and must be deprived of the seeds before use.

Fructus Colocynthidis præparati.

[PREPARED COLOCYNTH]. Präparirte Koloquinten.

Take of Colocynth, deprived of seeds, and finely cut,
five parts, ... 5
Gum Arabic, powdered, *one part*. . . . 1

With sufficient Distilled Water make a paste, which, when dry, reduce to a fine powder, and preserve it *cautiously* in a well-closed vessel.

It forms a yellowish powder, which has a very bitter taste.

Fructus Coriandri.

[CORIANDER SEEDS]. Koriandersamen.

[*Coriander Fruit*]. *Semen Coriandri.*

Coriandrum sativum *Linn.*

The fruit is globose, hollow, crowned with the calyx, two to three millimetres in diameter, and of a yellowish-brown color. The mericarps are mostly coherent, numerously striated on the back, and without vittæ. The taste of coriander is sweetish, burning when chewed, and the odor is aromatic.

Fructus Fœniculi.

[FENNEL SEEDS]. Fenchelsamen.

[*Fennel Fruit*]. *Semen Fœniculi.*

Fœniculum officinale *Allione* (**Anethum Fœniculum** *Linn.*)

The fruit is oblong, somewhat terete, of a brownish, or greenish color, about four millimetres long; mericarps easily separable; with five pale, keeled ribs; channels brown, in each a single vitta. They have a somewhat sweetish taste, burning when chewed, and a peculiar odor.

Fructus Juniperi.

[JUNIPER BERRIES]. Wachholderbeeren.

Baccæ Juniperus.

Juniperus communis ***Linn.***

The berries are globose, about the size of a pea, fleshy, trigibbous at the top, three-seeded; externally black, and covered with a bluish-green bloom; the flesh is of a greenish-brown color; the seeds are osseous, and glandular. The berries have a sweetish taste at first, afterwards somewhat bitter; their odor is aromatic.

Juniper Berries that are unripe, green, gray, or brownish-red, and those that are too old, must be rejected.

Fructus Lauri.

[BAY BERRIES]. Lorbeeren.

Baccæ Lauri.

Laurus nobilis ***Linn.***

The dried drupes are oval, wrinkled, and of a brownish-black color, about the size of a small cherry; the mesocarp is thin; putamen brownish-red and papery; seeds consisting of two fleshy, oleaginous, easily separable, nearly hemispherical cotyledons, of a brownish color. Their odor is peculiar, and their taste oily and bitter.

Fructus Myrtilli.

[MYRTLE BERRIES]. Heidelbeeren.

[***Whortleberries. Bilberries***]. ***Baccæ Myrtilli.***

Vaccinium Myrtillus ***Linn.***

Berries globular, umbilicate, many-seeded, dry, wrinkled, and of the size of a pea, with a black color; filled with a bluish-purple pulp, having a sweet-acidulous and mildly astringent taste. The berries should be sufficiently soft, not worm-eaten, or mouldy.

Fructus Papaveris.

[POPPY HEADS]. Mohnköpfe.

Capita vel Capsulæ Papaveris.

Papaver somniferum *Linn.*

The immature capsules [heads], about the size of a walnut, ovate-oblong; crowned with the large, radiate, peltate stigma; provided with numerous, parietal sporophores [placentæ], and many dry seeds. Poppy heads have a nauseous, bitter taste.

Fructus Petroselini.

[PARSLEY SEEDS]. Petersiliensamen.

[*Parsley Fruit*]. *Semen Petroselini.*

Petroselinum sativum *Hoffman.*

The fruit is ovate, compressed on the sides, about two millimetres long, smooth, and of a grayish-green color; mericarps easily separable; with five filiform ribs; channels elevated in the middle, each one with a single vitta. The fruit has a slightly burning taste, and a strong odor.

Fructus Phellandrii.

[FINE-LEAVED WATER-HEMLOCK SEEDS]. Wasserfenchel.

Semen Phellandrii aquatici.

Œnanthe Phellandrium *Lamarck.*

The fruit is oblong, subterate, narrowing towards the top, crowned with the calyx, about four millimetres long, and of a brown color. The mericarps are generally coherent, with five obtuse ribs; channels narrow, with single vittæ. Their odor is disagreeably aromatic, and their taste bitterish. The fruit should be perfectly ripe.

It should not be confounded with the fruits of *Cicuta virosa* Linn., and *Sium latifolium* Linn., which are recognized by their subglobose or ovate form, and their greenish color.

Fructus Rhamni catharticæ.

[BUCKTHORN BERRIES]. Kreuzdornbeeren.

Baccæ Spinæ cervinæ. Baccæ Rhamni catharticæ.

Rhamnus cathartica *Linn.*

The recent mature drupes; globose, about eight millimetres in thickness, supported by an orbicular disk [base of the calyx]. The drupes are black, and filled with a greenish-violet juice; they contain mostly four cartilaginous, obtusely three-cornered nutlets (pyrenæ), which are one-seeded and grooved (campylospermous). The drupe of Alder Buckthorn (*Rhamnus Frangula* Linn.), contains two or three nutlets, which are flat (orthospermous), and of a pale brownish color.

Fructus Sabadillæ.

[CEVADILLA SEEDS]. Sabadillsamen.

Semen Sabadillæ.

Sabadilla officinalis *Brandt.*

The carpels are in the form of three capsules united, papery, light-brown, opening at the ventral suture, many-seeded, and about twelve millimetres long, with the seeds generally fallen out. The seeds are elongated, angular, narrowing upwards, of a brownish-black color, internally white, four to six millimetres long, having an exceedingly bitter and very acrid, persistent taste.

Cevadilla seeds should be *cautiously* preserved.

Fructus Vanillæ.

[VANILLA]. Vanille.

Siliqua Vanillæ.

Vanilla planifolia *Andrews.*

The not fully ripe, dry capsules (pods), somewhat fleshy, pressed in a triangular shape, tapering toward both extremities, striated, flexible, and frequently covered with minute crystals. They are from one and a half to two and a half decimetres long, and from four to eight millimetres wide, of a dark-brown color, one-celled, and closely filled with a granular pulp, which has a very agreeable taste, and an odor resembling that of Balsam of Peru, and consists of innumerable, exceedingly small black seeds, which are agglutinated and covered with a very thin, balsamic layer.

Very unripe, slender, or juiceless fruit should not be employed, nor if already opened at the two valves; neither the fruit that occurs in commerce as Laguayra and Pompona Vanilla, which are thicker, but of a much feebler odor.

Fumigati Chlori.

[CHLORINE FUMIGATION]. Chlorräucherung.

For *stronger* fumigation, equal weights of Common Salt and Black Oxide of Manganese are mixed, and *two parts* of Crude Sulphuric Acid, previously diluted with *one part* of water poured upon them.

For *milder* fumigation, Vinegar is added to Chlorinated Lime, previously made into a paste with water.

Fungus igniarius præparatus.

[AGARIC OF THE OAK]. Feuerschwamm.

[*Spunk. Surgeon's Agaric*]. *Boletus igniarius vel Chirurgorum.*

Polyporus fomentarius *Fries.*

In very soft, rust-brown slices, deprived of the hard rind and hymenium. They must not have been treated with nitrate of potassium.

Fungus Laricis.

[LARCH AGARIC]. Lärchenschwamm.

[*White Agaric. Purging Agaric*]. *Agaricus albus. Boletus Laricis.*

Polyporus officinalis *Fries* (**Boletus Laricis** *Linn.*)

In light, spongy, fibrous pieces, which are friable, but tough, and not easily pulverized. They have a yellowish-white color, and a sweetish taste at first, afterwards bitter and acrid.

The decorticated agaric is only employed; the worm-eaten, however, must be rejected.

Galbanum.

[GALBANUM]. Mutterharz.

Gummi-resina Galbanum.

Ferula erubescens *Boissier.*

Either in distinct, or in agglutinated tears, of irregular shape, from the size of a pea to that of a hazelnut, having a pale-yellow, reddish- or brownish-yellow color. Their fracture has a waxy lustre, and a yellowish color. Sometimes it consists of more or less soft, greenish, or pale-brown lumps, having a lighter or darker marbled fracture.

Galbanum has an acrid and bitter taste, and a strongly balsamic odor.

It is powdered in cold weather, and separated from impurities by means of a sieve.

Gallæ.

[NUTGALL. GALLS]. Galläpfel.

Gallæ Halepenses v. Levanticæ v. Turcicæ.

Quercus infectoria *Olivier.*

Excrescences produced by the puncture of the gall-fly, *Cynips Gallæ tinctoriæ*, on the leaf-bud of a species of a shrubby, evergreen oak, growing in the East. Galls are more or less globular, and covered with sharp, warty protuberances; they are heavy, hard, and often exhibit a circular hole. They have a greenish-gray color, varying from a lighter to a darker shade, and an astringent taste when chewed.

The light, spongy, smooth—the so-called German galls—should be rejected.

Gelatina.

[GELATINE]. Weisser Leim.

[*White Glue*].

It should be almost colorless and inodorous.

Gelatina Carrageen.

[CARRAGEEN JELLY]. Irländisch-Moosgallerte.
Karrageengallerte.

Take of Irish Moss *one part*, ... 1
Common Water *forty parts*, ... 40
boil for half an hour by the heat of a steam-bath, and strain by expression. Then add of
Best White Sugar *two parts*, ... 2
and evaporate the whole, stirring constantly, to *ten parts*. 10

It is prepared only when wanted for dispensing.

Gelatina Lichenis Islandici.

[ICELAND MOSS JELLY]. Isländisch-Moosgallerte.

Take of Iceland Moss, washed in cold water, *three parts*, 3
Common Water *one hundred parts*, . . . 100
boil for half an hour by means of a steam-bath, and strain by expression. To the strained liquid, add of
Best White Sugar *three parts*, ... 3
and evaporate the whole, stirring constantly, to *ten parts*. 10

It is prepared only when wanted for dispensing.

Gelatina Lichenis Islandici saccharata sicca.

[DRY SACCHARATED ICELAND MOSS JELLY]. Trockne gezuckerte Isländisch-Moosgallerte.

Take of Iceland Moss, cut, *sixteen parts*, . . . 16
Purified Carbonate of Potassium *one part*. . 1

Pour sufficient Common Water upon them so that they shall be covered, then set aside for twenty-four hours, and stir occasionally. Having poured off the liquid, diligently wash the moss with common water, until the bitter and alkaline taste is removed. Then pour upon the washed moss
Common Water *two hundred parts*, . . . 200
and boil for four hours, by means of a steam-bath, stirring occasionally, and strain. Repeat the boiling of the moss with a fresh quantity of water. Strain the liquids, and add of
Best White Sugar *six parts*, ... 6
and boil until the mass is no longer sticky. It is then pulled to pieces and dried. The dried mass is weighed, and an amount of sugar added sufficient to make the sugar and the dried jelly equal in weight.

It is a grayish-brown powder, and has a sweet, mucilaginous, afterwards bitterish, taste.

Gemmæ Populi.

[POPLAR-BUDS]. Pappelknospen.

Oculi Populi.

Populus nigra *Linn.*, and other species of Populus.

The buds are conical, invested with sticky, resinous, imbricated scales (tegments). They have a pleasant odor. The buds are gathered in spring, before they open, and are employed in the recent state, or dried for future use.

Glandulæ Lupuli.

[LUPULIN]. Hopfenmehl.

Lupulin.

Humulus Lupulus *Linn.*

A somewhat resinous powder, of a golden-yellow color, changing by age to a yellowish-brown; consisting of very small, top-shaped, at the vertex roundish, glands; filled with a lemon-yellow balsam of a peculiar odor and bitter taste. The glands are separated from the recently dried strobiles of the hop by means of a hair-sieve. They must not be kept over a year, and must be free from sand.

Glycerinum.

[GLYCERIN]. Glycerin.

A transparent, colorless, inodorous syrupy liquid, of a sweet taste. It is neutral to test-paper, and has a specific gravity varying from 1.23 to 1.25. Soluble in all proportions of water, alcohol, and spirit of ether. Insoluble in ether, chloroform, and the fixed oils. The aqueous solution is not rendered turbid by oxalate of ammonium, or hydrosulphuric acid. Heated with solution of caustic potassa, it is not colored brown, nor should this alkaline mixture turn red on the addition of sulphate of copper. When heated with diluted sulphuric acid, and evaporated, the liquid is not colored black. Mixed with alcohol and concentrated sulphuric acid, it must not give off the odor of butyric ether. Glycerin should not separate metallic silver from a solution of nitrate of silver, to which has been added water of ammonia.

Gummi Arabicum.

[GUM ARABIC]. Arabisches Gummi.

Gummi Mimosæ.

Acacia Nilotica *Delile.* **Acacia Seyal** *Delile.* **Acacia tortilis** *Hayne.*

In irregular, rounded or angular pieces of various size. They are translucent, colorless, or slightly yellowish; finely and numerously fissured. They have a small conchoidal, glassy fracture, which is often iridescent. Gum Arabic becomes mucilaginous when chewed. It is insipid and inodorous.

It forms readily a mucilage with water, which becomes turbid on the addition of alcohol.

Gutta Percha depurata.

[PURIFIED GUTTA PERCHA]. Guttapercha.

Gutta Tuban.

Isonandra Gutta *Hooker.*

Occurring in a white or yellowish-white mass, sometimes streaked with a red coloring matter, formed into rolls of four or five centimetres in thickness, which are nearly inelastic, but flexible. It becomes soft and plastic at a heat of between 65° and 70° C., and melts at the temperature of boiling water. It is insoluble in water, partially soluble in alcohol, and ether, entirely so in the essential oils, bisulphide of carbon, and chloroform. It should be preserved under water.

Gutti.

[GAMBOGE]. Gutti.

Gummigutt. Gummi-resina Gutti.

Garcinia Morella *Desrousseaux,* (**Garcinia Gutta** *Wight*).

Mostly in cylindrical, brittle rolls, of an orange-yellow color, with a broadly conchoidal fracture, which is smooth, and of a waxy lustre; the edges of the broken pieces are somewhat translucent, and the powder has a lemon-yellow color. It is inodorous, and tasteless at first, afterwards sweetish, and causes a burning sensation in the mouth. Gamboge is partially dissolved by alcohol and ether. It produces, when rubbed with water, a light-yellow emulsion, and forms with a dilute solution of caustic potassa, or carbonate of potassium, a dark orange-yellow solution, from which the resin, of a lemon-yellow color, is precipitated by acids.

It should be *cautiously* preserved.

Herba Absinthii.

[WORMWOOD]. Wermuth.

Summitates Absinthii.

Artemisia Absinthium *Linn.*

The herb with the flowering panicle; the leaves are whitish-gray, silky, pinnately two or three-cleft; the terminal segments spatulate; the upper leaves are undivided. The flower-heads are subglobose, nodding, with a villose receptacle, and small, yellowish florets. Wormwood has a very bitter taste, and a strong aromatic odor.

It should be gathered in July and August, and be separated from the larger stems.

Herba Cannabis Indicæ.

[INDIAN HEMP]. Indischer Hanf.

Cannabis sativa *Linn.*

The flowering branches of the female plant, being partially in fruit, covered with appressed hairs, and rough to the touch. It occurs in the form of compressed, dense bundles or whisps, of the leafy flowering tops, agglutinated by the exudation of a resin. The floral leaves are entire, lanceolate, linear, serrate. The calyx is bract-like, vaginate, inclosing the female flower, and later the well-known fruit, and is covered with brownish-red glands. Indian Hemp has a peculiar narcotic odor, especially when warmed.

That which is grown in India only should be used.

Herba Cardui benedicti.

[BLESSED THISTLE]. Kardobenediktenkraut.

Folia Cardui benedicti.

Cnicus benedictus *Linn.*

Leaves about two decimetres in length, lanceolate or oblong-lanceolate, narrowing to the petiole, sinuately pinnatifid, acutely dentate, hairy, and of a very bitter, saline taste.

The herb with the flowers should be gathered.

Herba Centaurii.

[European Centaury]. Tausendguldenkraut.

Herba Centaurii minoris.

Erythræa Centaurium *Persoon* (**Gentiana Centaurium** *Linn.*).

The flowering herb; stem angular, simple at the base, and cymo-corymbosely branched above. The leaves are opposite, sessile, oblong-oval or narrow, three to five nerved and entirely smooth. Corolla red; anthers spirally twisted after flowering. European Centaury has a bitter taste.

It should be gathered in July and August.

Herba Chelidonii.

[Celandine]. Schöllkraut.

Chelidonium majus *Linn.*

The entire fresh herb is filled with a saffron-colored, bitter, acrid juice. Branches jointed, slightly hairy; leaves almost lyrate, beneath bluish-green, pubescent, particularly at the nerves, with roundish, crenate lobes. Flowers yellow, with four petals, in umbel-like clusters.

It should be gathered in May.

Herba Chenopodii ambrosioidis.

[Mexican Tea-Plant]. Mexikanisches Traubenkraut.

[*Mexican Tea*]. *Jesuitenthee. Herba Botryos Mexicanæ.*

Chenopodium ambrosioides *Linn.*

The flowering herb; the leaves are scattered, oblong or lanceolate, tapering to both ends, remotely dentate, smooth, of a bright-green color, glandular beneath. The flowers are apetalous, very small, and arranged in axillary glomerules. It produces a burning sensation in the mouth when chewed, and has a bitter taste, and a strong balsamic odor.

It should be gathered in July.

Herba Cochleariæ.

[COMMON SCURVY-GRASS]. Löffelkraut.

Cochlearia officinalis *Linn.*

The fresh flowering herb; radical leaves petiolate, roundish, subcordate, repand, mostly wanting; cauline leaves almost clasping, ovate, sinuate-toothed. The flowers are white and the silicles turgid. The rubbed herb exhales a volatile acrid odor. It has a bitter burning taste.

It should be gathered in the spring.

Herba Conii.

[CONIUM LEAVES]. Schierlingskraut.

[*Hemlock. Common or Spotted Hemlock. Poison Hemlock*]. *Herba Conii maculati. Herba Cicutæ.*

Conium maculatum *Linn.*

The flowering herb, smooth throughout, with decompound leaves, which have a sheathing base, and the lower ones hollow petioles; the upper ones are sessile, and nearly opposite; terminal segments oval-oblong, incised-serrate and mucronate. Flowers umbellate, small, white, with nearly globular ovaries, and more or less unripe fruits, furnished with crenulated ridges (ribs). The herb has a peculiarly nauseous odor. The genuine plant is readily distinguished from other allied species of Umbelliferæ, such as *Anthriscus silvestris* Hofm., *Chærophyllum hirsutum, bulbosum, temulum* L., *Æthusa Cynapium* L., *Cicuta virosa* L., &c., by means of a magnifying glass, when the crenulate ridges (ribs) of the ovary or unripe fruit are discernible, and also by its peculiar odor, when the dried leaves are moistened with solution of caustic potassa. It is distinguished from species of *Anthriscus* and *Chærophyllum* by the entire smoothness of the hemlock.

Hemlock leaves should be gathered in summer from plants with brown or red-spotted stems, be separated from the larger branches, and *cautiously* preserved, but should not be kept longer than a year.

The powder should be prepared from the recently dried leaves, and be *cautiously* preserved in well-closed vessels, and in a dark place.

Herba Galeopsidis.

[HEMP-NETTLE]. Hohlzahn.

Blankenheimer Thee. Lieber'sché Kräuter.

Galeopsis ochroleuca *Lamarck.*

The flowering herb, with a four-angled stem, softly pubescent, not swollen below the joints (nodes); the leaves are opposite, petiolate, ovate-oblong; upper ones oblong, somewhat silky-pubescent on both sides and of a yellowish-green color. The flowers are large, arranged in axillary whorls (verticillasters), which are more distant below. Corolla bilabiate, yellowish-white, externally hairy, four times the length of the spiny-tipped, toothed calyx. The herb has a faint odor, and a saline, bitterish taste.

Care should be taken that it be not confounded with *Galeopsis Ladanum* L., having lanceolate or oblong-lanceolate leaves, and small purple flowers; nor with *Galeopsis versicolor* Curt., with a bristly-hairy stem, swollen below the joints.

Herba Gratiolæ.

[HEDGE HYSSOP]. Gottesgnadenkraut.

Gratiola officinalis *Linn.*

The smooth flowering herb, with a stiff, four-angled stem, branching above. Leaves opposite, sessile, lanceolate, remotely serrate, three to five-nerved. Flowers solitary, axillary, with a bibracteolate peduncle, and a sublabiate, white corolla. Hedge Hyssop produces a burning sensation in the mouth when chewed, and has a bitter, nauseous taste.

It should be gathered in June and July, and must be *cautiously* preserved.

Herba Lactucæ.

[ACRID, OR STRONG-SCENTED LETTUCE]. Giftlattich.

Herba Lactucæ virosæ.

Lactuca virosa *Linn.*

The fresh, milky, panicled herb. Leaves horizontal, with sagittate, clasping base, oblong, entire or sinuate, with mucronate teeth; prickly on the midrib. Flower-heads radiate, few-flowered, yellow. The plant has a disagreeable, narcotic odor, and an unpleasant, bitter, saline taste. It should not be confounded with *Lactuca Scariola* Linn., which is known by its sinuate-pinnatifid, vertical leaves.

The biennial herb, with the flowering branches, should be gathered, either from the wild-growing plant, particularly that found in Western Europe, or from the cultivated herb, and should be made into extract in its recent state.

Herba Linariæ.

[COMMON TOAD-FLAX]. Leinkraut.

Herba cum floribus Linariæ.

Linaria vulgaris ***Miller.***

The fresh flowering herb, with scattered, crowded leaves, which are sessile, linear, pointed, entire, smooth, and three-nerved. Flowers in a raceme, yellow, personate, spurred at their base.

The leafy, flowering tops should be gathered in summer.

Herba Lobeliæ.

[LOBELIA]. Lobelienkraut.

[***Indian Tobacco***]. ***Herba Lobeliæ inflatæ.***

Lobelia inflata ***Linn.***

The flowering herb; somewhat hairy; leaves scattered, lower ones with short petioles, oblong, unequally toothed. Flowers in racemes, small, epigynous; segments of the calyx linear, equalling in length the corolla, which is bilabiate, and of a pale violet color; capsule inflated. The herb has a mild taste at first, which becomes acrid when chewed.

Lobelia cultivated in Germany may be employed, but should be freed from the larger stems.

Herba Majoranæ.

[SWEET MARJORAM]. Meiran.

Origanum Majorana ***Linn.***

The flowering herb; paniculate, hoary-tomentose; leaves opposite, oval or oblong, obtuse and entire. Spikes with four rows of imbricated, roundish bracts. Marjoram has an aromatic odor.

The plant should be gathered in summer.

Herba Meliloti.

[MELILOT]. Steinklee.

Melilotenklee. Summitates Meliloti.

Melilotus officinalis ***Persoon.***

The flowering branches with ternate leaves and awl-shaped stipules. Corolla papilionaceous, small, yellow, with ovary and fruit covered with silky hairs. Melilot has a peculiar odor.

The branches of the biennial plant should be gathered in July and August.

Herba Millefolii.

[YARROW]. Schafgarbenkraut.

[***Milfoil***]. ***Folia Millefolii.***

Achillea Millefolium ***Linn.***

Doubly pinnate leaves; lanceolate in their outline; villose on the petioles and nerves of their lower surface. The segments are decurrent, lanceolate, acuminate, mucronate, and glandular beneath. Yarrow has a bitter taste.

It should be collected in June.

Herba Polygalæ.

[BITTER MILKWORT]. Kreuzblumenkraut.

[***European Bitter Polygala***]. ***Herba Polygalæ amaræ.***

Polygala amara ***Linn.***

The flowering plant; growing in a tufted form (cæspitose), with slender yellow roots. The numerous stems rise to the height of about ten centimetres. The lower leaves are the larger, spatulate or obovate, and disposed in a rosette; the upper ones scattered, lanceolate. The flowers are small, blue or white, racemose. Two of the (five) sepals are winged-shaped and petaloid. The plant has a very bitter taste.

It should not be confounded with other species of Polygala, from which it is distinguished, particularly, by its rosulate leaves and its very bitter taste.

It should be collected in May and July.

Herba Pulsatillæ.

[PULSATILLA]. Küchenschelle.

[*Meadow Anemone and Pulsatilla Anemone*]. *Herba Pulsatillæ nigricantis.*

Anemone pratensis and Anemone Pulsatilla *Linn.*

The fresh flowering herb; clothed with soft hairs, having pinnately two to three-cleft radical leaves, with linear segments; the leaves are not developed at the time of flowering; scape one-flowered; involucre foliaceous, many parted, distant from the dark-violet or sky-blue, campanulate flower. The whole herb is inodorous, but exhales, by rubbing, a very acrid vapor, and when chewed produces a violent burning.

It should be collected in April and May.

Herba Serpylli.

[WILD THYME]. Quendel.

[*Mother of Thyme*]. *Feldkümmelkraut. Wilder Thymian.*

Thymus Serpyllum *Linn.*

The flowering herb; with a thin prostrate stem. Leaves opposite, small, flat, varying from narrow to broad, glandular on both sides, ciliate at their base. Flowers in subcapitate whorls, with corolla and calyx bilabiate. The plant has a fragrant odor and a somewhat bitter, astringent taste.

It should be gathered in summer.

Herba Spilanthis.

[SPEARLEAVED SPILANTHUS]. Parakresse.

Herba Spilanthis oleraceæ.

Spilanthes oleracea *Jacquin.*

The flowering herb; with a branching stem; leaves opposite, petiolate, oval, subcordate, repand-crenate, three-nerved, margin scabrous. Peduncles axillary, solitary, longer than the leaves, each with one flower-head, which is discoid, dense, ovate, having numerous florets, first brown, changing to yellow.

When the herb is chewed it produces a burning sensation in the mouth, and a copious flow of saliva.

Herba Thymi.

[THYME]. Gartenthymian.

Römischer Quendel.

Thymus vulgaris *Linn.*

The flowering herb with a slender, erect, puberulent stem. Leaves opposite, small, oblong, with revolute margins, not ciliate, glandular on both sides, beneath hoary-puberulent. Whorls axillary, the upper ones crowded. Calyx and corolla bilabiate. Thyme has a fragrant odor.

Herba Violæ tricoloris.

[PANSY]. Freisamkraut.

[***Heartsease***]. ***Stiefmütterchenthee.*** ***Herba Jaceæ.***

Viola tricolor *Linn.*

The flowering herb; stem angular; leaves scattered, petiolate, oblong, crenate; stipules lyrate, longer than the petiole. Flowers axillary with long peduncles. Corolla labiate, spurred, two to three-colored, or yellowish. When chewed somewhat burning, with a bitterish taste.

The herb with light-blue flowers should have the preference. The cultivated must be rejected.

Hirudines.

[LEECH]. Blutegel.

Sanguisuga medicinalis et Sanguisuga officinalis ***Savigny.***

The first species, called the German Leech, is rough-grained, above [back] of an olive-green color, with six pale, rusty-red, longitudinal stripes, which are spotted with black. Beneath [belly] it is greenish-yellow, marked with black spots and black margins. The other species, known as Hungarian Leech, is smooth; above greenish or blackish green, with six rusty-red, black-spotted, longitudinal stripes; beneath of an olive-green, unspotted, but marked with a black stripe on each side.

Those previously employed are to be rejected.

The horse-leech, *Hæmopis* (*Hippobdella* Blainville), *Sanguisorba* Savigny, is inappropriate for use, and is distinguished by its irregular spots on the back, without stripes.

Hydrargyrum.

[Mercury]. Quecksilber.

[*Quicksilver*]. *Mercurius vivus.*

A liquid, bluish-white metal, of a metallic lustre, and usually containing small quantities of lead, bismuth, tin, and zinc.

Hydrargyrum bichloratum corrosivum.

[Corrosive Chloride of Mercury]. Aetzendes Quecksilberchlorid.

[*Bichloride of Mercury. Perchloride of Mercury. Corrosive Sublimate*]. *Aetzender Quecksilbersublimat. Mercurius sublimatus corrosivus.*

In white, translucent, heavy, crystalline masses, of a radiated structure and granular fracture. It melts when heated, and is afterwards entirely volatilized. It dissolves in sixteen parts of cold, and in three parts of boiling water; also soluble in three parts of alcohol, and in four parts of cold ether.

It should be *very cautiously* preserved in well-closed vessels.

Hydrargyrum biiodatum rubrum.

[Red Iodide of Mercury]. Rothes Quecksilberjodid.

[*Biniodide of Mercury*]. *Rothes Jodquecksilber. Mercurius iodatus ruber. Deutoioduretum Hydrargyri.*

Take of Corrosive Chloride of Mercury *four parts*, . 4
dissolve it in
Distilled Water *seventy-two parts*. . . . 72
Then dissolve
Iodide of Potassium *five parts*, ... 5
in
Distilled Water *sixteen parts*. 16

Filter both solutions and mix them with agitation. Collect the resulting precipitate on a filter, and having washed it thoroughly with distilled water, dry it.

It forms a very fine, bright scarlet powder, very sparingly soluble in water, wholly soluble in alcohol. Exposed to heat it volatilizes without leaving a residue.

It should be *very cautiously* preserved in well-closed vessels.

Hydrargyrum chloratum mite.

[MILD CHLORIDE OF MERCURY]. Quecksilberchlorür.

[*Subchloride of Mercury. Calomel*]. *Calomel. Hydrargyrum chloratum mite lævigatum. Hydrargyrum muriaticum mite. Mercurius dulcis. Calomelas.*

It is prepared by sublimation. A very fine, heavy, yellowish-white powder; insoluble in water or alcohol. Infusible, but wholly volatilizable by heat. It is blackened when mixed with a solution of caustic potassa or soda, but yields no ammoniacal odor. When shaken with ten times its weight of cold water or alcohol, and filtered, the filtrate should not be affected by hydrosulphuric acid. It is soluble in nitric acid of the specific gravity 1.4, with evolution of a yellowish-red vapor.

It should be *cautiously* preserved in vessels protected from the light.

Hydrargyrum chloratum mite vapore paratum.

[MILD CHLORIDE OF MERCURY PREPARED BY STEAM].
Durch Dampf bereitetes Quecksilberchlorür.

Calomelas vapore paratum.

A very soft, white powder, which, when rather strongly triturated in a porcelain mortar, assumes a yellow color, but behaves in other respects like calomel prepared by sublimation.

It should be *cautiously* preserved, and kept in a dark place.

Hydrargyrum depuratum.

[PURIFIED MERCURY]. Gereinigtes Quecksilber.

Take of Mercury *one hundred parts*, ...	100
Nitric Acid, ...	5
Distilled Water, each, *five parts*, ...	5

Introduce them into a suitable glass vessel, and digest for three days, shaking frequently. Having poured off the acid liquid, wash well the mercury with distilled water, and dry it completely by means of a steam-bath.

When the metal is exposed to a strong heat it is dissipated, leaving no residue.

Hydrargyrum iodatum flavum.

[GREEN IODIDE OF MERCURY, U. S. P.]. Quecksilberjodür.

[*Iodide of Mercury. Protiodide of Mercury*]. *Gelbes Jodquecksilber. Hydrargyrum iodatum. Protoioduretum Hydrargyri.*

Take of Purified Mercury *eight parts*, ...	8
Iodine *five parts*.	5

Triturate, gradually, the iodine in a porcelain mortar with the mercury, moistening the mixture with a few drops of alcohol, until no more globules of mercury are visible, and the mixture has assumed a greenish-yellow color. Then wash the mass with alcohol, and dry it in a warm place.

In the form of a fine, heavy, greenish-yellow powder, which becomes brown when exposed to the light. It is insoluble in ether, sparingly soluble in water, and scarcely so in alcohol. It is wholly volatilized by heat. Alcohol, when well shaken with the powder, and separated by filtration, is scarcely altered by hydrosulphuric acid.

It should be *very cautiously* preserved, and protected from the light.

Hydrargyrum nitricum oxydulatum.

[SUBNITRATE OF MERCURY]. Salpetersaures Quecksilberoxydul.

[*Mercurous nitrate.*]

In small, colorless crystals, which cannot be dissolved in water without decomposing the salt; but it is completely soluble in water, acidulated with nitric acid. It yields with lime-water a grayish-black precipitate. The solution, formed by the action of nitric acid, and wholly precipitated by hydrochloric acid, and filtered, is not altered by protochloride of tin, or hydrosulphuric acid.

It should be *very cautiously* preserved in well-closed vessels.

Hydrargyrum oxydatum rubrum.

[RED OXIDE OF MERCURY]. Rothes Quecksilberoxyd.

[*Red Precipitate*]. *Rother Quecksilberpräcipitat. Mercurius præcipitatus ruber.*

A very fine, heavy, lustreless, yellowish-red powder; volatilized by heat without the evolution of yellowish-red vapors. Completely soluble in hydrochloric or nitric acid; not affected by oxalic acid.

It should be *very cautiously* preserved, and protected from the light.

Hydrargyrum oxydatum via humida paratum.

[PRECIPITATED RED OXIDE OF MERCURY]. Präcipitirtes Quecksilberoxyd.

Take of Corrosive Chloride of Mercury *one part*. . . 1
Dissolve it in
Hot Distilled Water *six parts*, ... 6
pour this solution, while stirring constantly, into a
Boiling Solution of Caustic Soda *one part*, . 1
which has been previously diluted with
Distilled Water *six parts*. 6

Separate the resulting precipitate, wash it well with boiling water, and dry it with a gentle heat.

A very soft, heavy, reddish-yellow powder, which is nearly wholly volatilized by heat. It turns white when mixed with a solution of oxalic acid.

It is dispensed only when expressly prescribed.

It should be *very cautiously* preserved, and protected from the light.

Hydrargyrum præcipitatum album.

[AMMONIATED MERCURY]. Weisser Quecksilberpräcipitat.

[*White Precipitate*]. ***Hydrargyrum amidato-bichloratum. Hydrargyrum ammoniato-muriaticum. Mercurius præcipitatus albus.***

Take of Corrosive Chloride of Mercury *two parts*. . . 2
Dissolve it in
Hot Distilled Water *forty parts*. 40
Pour the cold, filtered solution, while stirring, into
Water of Ammonia *three parts*, ... 3
or so much that it shall be in slight excess; then collect the resulting precipitate in a filter, allow it to drain as much as possible, and wash it twice, each time with
Distilled Water *eighteen parts*, ... 18
and afterwards dry it in a dark place.

A very white powder; insoluble in water, but readily soluble in hot nitric acid. It is colored yellow, with evolution of ammonia, when heated with solution of caustic soda. It is entirely volatilized by heat, without fusing.

It should be *very cautiously* preserved in well-closed vessels, and protected from the light.

Hydrargyrum sulfuratum nigrum.

[BLACK SULPHURET OF MERCURY]. Schwarzes Schwefelquecksilber.

[*Ethiops Mineral*]. ***Æthiops mineralis.***

Take of Purified Mercury,
Washed Flowers of Sulphur, each, *equal parts*.

Rub them together at a moderate heat, until they are converted into a uniform black powder, in which no globules of mercury can be detected with the aid of a lens.

A very fine, black, heavy powder; insoluble in water, alcohol, hydrochloric or nitric acid. When heated it burns with a blue flame, leaving no residue. Digested with hydrochloric acid, and filtered, the filtrate is not affected by hydrosulphuric acid.

Hydrargyrum sulfuratum rubrum.

[RED SULPHURET OF MERCURY]. Zinnober.

[*Sulphide of Mercury. Cinnabar. Vermilion*]. *Cinnabaris.*

A bright red powder, burning when exposed to heat with a blue flame, evolving vapors of sulphurous acid, and leaving no residue. It is insoluble in water, alcohol, hydrochloric acid, or nitric acid; insoluble also in a diluted solution of caustic potassa or soda, but soluble in cold nitro-muriatic acid.

Cinnabar, when shaken with nitric acid, does not change its color: if this mixture be gently heated and diluted with water, it yields a colorless filtrate, which is not colored black by the addition of hydrosulphuric acid. When well shaken with water and solution of caustic potassa or soda, and heated, the mixture yields a colorless filtrate, which is not altered by hydrochloric acid, but on the addition of acetate of lead it throws down a white precipitate.

Infusa.

[INFUSIONS]. Aufgüsse.

Infusions which are ordered without a given quantity of the substance to be used, are made so that from *one part* of substance *ten parts* of colature (strained infusion) are procured. To prepare *ten parts* of a colature of a *concentrated infusion, one and a half parts* of the substance are used; and to prepare *ten parts* of a colature of *a highly concentrated infusion, two parts* of the substance are taken.

The quantity of medicinally active substances must always be determined by the physician.

The substance is put in a suitable vessel, boiling water poured upon it, then covered and exposed to the heat of a steam-bath for five minutes. The vessel is then set aside, and the *cold* infusion is strained with expression.

Infusum Sennæ compositum.

[COMPOUND INFUSION OF SENNA]. Wiener Trank.

[*Vienna Black Draught*].

Take of Senna, cut, *two parts*, ... 2
Pour upon it
Boiling Water *twelve parts*, ... 12
and expose to the heat of a steam-bath for five minutes, stirring frequently. Then express, and dissolve in the colature
Tartarate of Potassium and Sodium *two parts*, 2
Common Manna *three parts*, ... 3
and strain. The colature should be *fifteen parts*. . . 15
It has a brown color.

Iodoformium.

[IODOFORM]. Jodoform.

In very small, crystalline plates, of a greasy feel, and lemon-yellow color, having the odor of saffron, and a disagreeable, iodine-like taste. It melts at from 115° to 120° C.; is volatile in boiling water, and entirely volatilized at a higher temperature. It is insoluble in water, but soluble in eighty parts of cold, and in twelve parts of boiling alcohol, and also in twenty parts of ether.

It should be *cautiously* preserved in a glass-stoppered bottle.

Iodum.

[IODINE]. Jod.

In heavy, grayish-black, crystalline scales, of a metallic lustre. They are dry and friable, having a peculiar odor. It is very slightly soluble in water, but dissolves in ten parts of alcohol, and freely in ether, chloroform, and bisulphide of carbon. A solution of starch is tinged a violet color by a very small quantity of iodine.

It should be *cautiously* preserved in glass-stoppered bottles.

Kali aceticum.

[ACETATE OF POTASSIUM]. Essigsaures Kali.

Terra foliata Tartari.

A very white, nearly neutral, crystalline powder. It is very deliquescent in the air; soluble in an equal part of water, and in four parts of alcohol.

An aqueous solution is not altered by hydrosulphuric acid, hydrosulphate of ammonium, or chloride of barium; and nitrate of silver renders it but slightly turbid.

It should be preserved in well-closed bottles.

Kali bicarbonicum.

[BICARBONATE OF POTASSIUM]. Saures oder doppelt-kohlensaures Kali.

In translucent, colorless crystals, permanent in the air, slowly soluble in four parts of water, and scarcely soluble in alcohol.

It is tested like pure carbonate of potassium.

Kali carbonicum crudum.

[CRUDE CARBONATE OF POTASSIUM]. Rohes kohlensaures Kali.

[Pearlash. Crude Potash]. Rohe Pottasche. Cineres clavellati.

A whitish salt, having generally a greenish or bluish tint. It has an acrid, alkaline taste, and is deliquescent in the air. The greater portion of it is soluble in an equal part of water.

It forms a dry powder, and if dissolved in an excess of hydrochloric acid, the solution is not altered by hydrosulphuric acid. The salt does not communicate a yellow color to the flame of alcohol. It should contain no less than *sixty-five per cent.* of carbonate of potassium, nor more than *eighteen per cent.* of water.

Kali carbonicum depuratum.

[PURIFIED CARBONATE OF POTASSIUM]. Gereinigtes kohlensaures Kali.

[*Carbonate of Potassium*]. *Kali carbonicum e cineribus clavellatis.*

A dry, white, granular powder, almost wholly soluble in an equal part of water.

Its aqueous solution, mixed with an excess of hydrochloric acid, must not be altered by hydrosulphuric acid, and be rendered but slightly turbid on the addition of chloride of barium. It contains about *eighty per cent.* of carbonate of potassium, and from *fifteen* to *eighteen per cent.* of water. The anhydrous salt should contain no less than *ninety-two per cent.* of carbonate of potassium.

It should be preserved in well-closed vessels.

Kali carbonicum purum.

[PURE CARBONATE OF POTASSIUM]. Reines kohlensaures Kali.

[*Salt of Tartar*]. *Kali carbonicum e Tartaro. Sal Tartari.*

It is very white, wholly soluble in an equal part of water, forming a clear solution. A diluted solution, treated with an excess of nitric acid, must not be affected by hydrosulphuric acid, or nitrate of barium, and should be rendered but slightly turbid by nitrate of silver.

It should be preserved in well-closed vessels.

Kali causticum fusum.

[CAUSTIC POTASSA]. Aetzkali.

[*Potassa, U. S. P.*] *Aetzstein. Kali hydricum fusum. Lapis causticus chirurgorum.*

In white, dry, brittle sticks, having a crystalline fracture.

It is very caustic; deliquescent in the air. When dissolved in double its weight of water, and then mixed with four times its weight of alcohol, it should yield but a very slight crystalline precipitate, or watery deposit. It should effervesce but little with nitric acid; and, when treated with an excess of sulphuric acid, the solution should not discharge the color of indigo solution. Otherwise it behaves, in the presence of reagents, like solution of caustic potassa.

It should be *cautiously* preserved.

Kali chloricum.

[Chlorate of Potassium]. Chlorsaures Kali.

Kali muriaticum oxygenatum.

In colorless, lamellar or tabular crystals, permanent in the air, and of a shining lustre. They dissolve in sixteen or seventeen parts of cold, and in three parts of boiling water.

Its aqueous solution should be rendered but slightly turbid by nitrate of silver.

Kali hypermanganicum crystallisatum.

[Permanganate of Potassium]. Uebermangansaures Kali.

In very dark-brown, acicular, or prismatic crystals, of a steel lustre. They dissolve in sixteen parts of cold, and in two parts of boiling water.

It should be preserved in glass-stoppered bottles.

Kali nitricum.

[Nitrate of Potassium]. Salpeter.

[*Saltpetre. Nitre*]. *Kalisalpeter. Nitrum depuratum.*

In transparent, colorless, prismatic crystals, permanent in the air; or in the form of a white crystalline powder. It is soluble in three parts of cold, and in less than half its weight of boiling water.

A dilute aqueous solution is not rendered turbid by chloride of barium, and only slightly so by nitrate of silver.

Kali sulfuricum.

[SULPHATE OF POTASSIUM]. Schwefelsaures Kali.

Tartarus vitriolatus depuratus. Arcanum duplicatum depuratum.

In hard, white, prismatic crystals, or in crystalline crusts; permanent in the air, even at an elevated temperature; soluble in nine parts of cold, and four parts of hot water.

The aqueous solution is neutral, and is not rendered turbid by hydrosulphate of ammonium, or carbonate of potassium.

Kali tartaricum.

[TARTRATE OF POTASSIUM]. Neutrales weinsaures Kali.

Tartarus tartarisatus.

In colorless, translucent crystals; soluble in three-fourths of a part of cold, and in half its weight of boiling water.

The aqueous solution is neutral, or scarcely alkaline; it is not altered by hydrosulphate or oxalate of ammonium; and, when acidulated by nitric acid, neither by hydrosulphuric acid nor chloride of barium; with nitrate of silver it becomes only slightly turbid.

It should be preserved in well-closed vessels.

Kalium bromatum.

[BROMIDE OF POTASSIUM]. Bromkalium.

Kali hydrobromicum.

In white, shining, cubic crystals; permanent in the air, and readily soluble in water, and alcohol.

It is not colored by diluted sulphuric acid. The aqueous solution, to which has been added, first a small quantity of fuming nitric acid, and then chloroform, must not communicate a violet color to the chloroform when the mixture is shaken. When distilled with a mixture of bichromate of potassium and sulphuric acid, it yields a red liquid (distillate), which is decolorized on the addition of water of ammonia in excess, but must in no case turn yellow, which would indicate the presence of chlorine.

Kalium ferrocyanatum.

[FERROCYANIDE OF POTASSIUM]. Ferrocyankalium.

[*Yellow Prussiate of Potash*]. *Blutlaugensalz. Ferro-Kalium cyanatum. Kali Borussicum.*

In large, yellow, prismatic, or short, four-sided, tabular crystals, adhering together in a mass. They do not effloresce in the air; dissolve in four parts of cold, and in two parts of hot water, but are insoluble in alcohol.

The salt does not effervesce on the addition of diluted sulphuric acid; but, on heating the acid mixture, it develops hydrocyanic acid. A highly diluted aqueous solution does not become turbid with chloride of barium.

Kalium jodatum.

[IODIDE OF POTASSIUM]. Jodkalium.

Kali hydroiodicum.

In colorless, cubic crystals, which do not become moist in dry air. They are soluble in three-fourths their weight of water, and in six parts of alcohol, giving a neutral, or very slightly alkaline solution.

The aqueous solution is not rendered turbid by lime-water, or chloride of barium, nor turned brown by diluted sulphuric acid.

The precipitate thrown down from the solution by nitrate of silver, then well washed and shaken with water of ammonia, yields a liquid which, when filtered, should only become turbid with a large excess of nitric acid, without yielding a precipitate.

It should be *cautiously* preserved in well-closed vessels.

Kalium sulfuratum.

[SULPHURET OF POTASSIUM]. Kalischwefelleber.

[*Liver of Sulphur*]. *Hepar Sulphuris ad usum internum.*

Take of Washed Sulphur *one part*, ... 1
Pure Carbonate of Potassium *two parts*. . . 2

Mix them intimately, expose the mixture in a porcelain vessel to a moderate heat until it ceases to swell, and is completely fused, and a small portion is found, on trial, to dissolve wholly in twice its weight of water. Then pour the mass into a porcelain mortar, and, either break it into pieces, or powder it coarsely, and introduce it immediately into a dry vessel, which must be well closed.

This preparation has a liver-brown color, changing to a greenish-yellow. It dissolves wholly in about two parts of water, and it is also soluble in alcohol.

Kalium sulfuratum ad balneum.

[SULPHURET OF POTASSIUM FOR BATHING]. Schwefelleber zum Bade.

Kali Sulphuratum pro balneo. Hepar Sulphuris pro balneo.

Take of Sulphur *one part*, ... 1
Dried Crude Carbonate of Potassium *two parts*. 2

Mix them, and expose the mixture, in a sufficiently capacious, covered, iron crucible, to a moderate heat, until it ceases to swell, and is converted into a uniform mass, which pour upon an iron plate, or into an iron mortar. It may then be broken in pieces, or coarsely powdered, and should be immediately introduced into vessels, which must be well closed.

It has a yellowish-green color, and dissolves in distilled water, leaving but a slight residue.

Kamala.

[KAMEELA. KAMALA]. Kamala.

Glandulæ Rottleræ.

Rottlera tinctoria *Roxburgh.*

A somewhat resinous powder, of a brownish-red or brick-red color, consisting of very small, depressed-roundish glands, which contain club-shaped vesicles, filled with a balsamic substance.

It should be as free as possible from minute, stellate hairs, with which it is generally mixed, and which are much lighter than the glands, and it should contain no sand.

Kino.

[KINO]. Kino.

Gummi vel Resina Kino.

Pterocarpus Marsupium *Martius.*

In small, irregular, angular, shining fragments, of a dark-brown color, with reddish translucent edges, very friable, yielding a red powder. It is inodorous, but has a very astringent taste. It swells in cold water, and becomes paler, but gives to the water a reddish color. It forms a turbid solution with hot water, and a dark-red with alcohol.

Kreosotum.

[CREASOTE]. Kreosot.

Buchenholztheerkreosot.

A clear, colorless liquid, changing to a yellowish or reddish color by age. It has a penetrating odor; boils at above 200° C.; is wholly soluble in eighty parts of cold, and in twenty-four parts of hot water. It dissolves also completely in all proportions of alcohol, ether, the oils, and in solution of caustic potassa.

It should not be miscible with water of ammonia, nor should a watery solution turn blue on the addition of solution of sesquichloride of iron.

It should be *cautiously* preserved.

Lactucarium.

[LACTUCARIUM]. Giftlattichsaft.

[***Lettuce Opium***]. ***Lactucarium Germanicum.***

Lactuca virosa *Linn.*

In irregular, dry and friable pieces, of a yellow or yellowish-brown color, with a waxy fracture, strongly narcotic odor, and a somewhat bitter taste. When triturated with water, it affords a turbid solution, and leaves a tough mass as a residue. Alcohol and also ether dissolve it partially.

It should be *cautiously* preserved.

Laminaria.

Laminaria Cloustoni ***Edmonston,*** (and partly **Laminaria digitata** ***Lamouroux***).

Consisting of stipes, from fifty to one hundred centimetres in length, and from one-half to one centimetre in thickness; cylindrical or slightly compressed, deeply furrowed, wrinkled, and horny. They are somewhat elastic, of a brown color, occasionally covered in the depressions of the wrinkles with a white salt, consisting of chloride of sodium. When macerated in water they assume an olive-green, or leek-green color, a cartilaginous consistence, and swell up to about four times their former thickness.

The thicker stipes are to be preferred.

Lichen Islandicus.

[ICELAND MOSS]. Isländisches Moos.

Isländische Flechte.

Cetraria Islandica ***Acharius,*** (**Lichen Islandicus** ***Linn.***)

Thallus erect, foliaceous, irregularly incised, with fringed and channeled lobes; brown on the upper [fertile] surface, paler beneath, and at the base of a blood-red color. When dry it is stiff, brittle; becoming soft when moistened, and somewhat leathery, having a bitter taste. A decoction gelatinizes on cooling.

Iceland Moss is frequently mixed with foreign Lichens, especially of the family of Cladoniaceæ, and also with various mosses, pine-leaves, and other impurities, which may be easily removed from the cut moss by means of a sieve.

Lichen Islandicus ab amaritie liberatus.

[ICELAND MOSS FREED FROM BITTERNESS]. Entbittertes Isländisches Moos.

Take of Iceland Moss, cut, *five parts*, ... 5

Pour upon it

Tepid Common Water *thirty parts*, ... 30

Solution of Carbonate of Potassa *one part*. . 1

Set aside for three hours, then, having poured off the liquid, wash the moss well with cold water.

Lignum Campechianum.

[LOGWOOD]. Blauholz.

Campecheholz.

Hæmatoxylon Campechianum *Linn.*

In large logs from the trunk of the tree, externally of a bluish-black color, and internally dark brownish-red. It is hard, heavy, showing large fibres on its split surface; and on the cross section, very close, wavy, concentric rings (layers), which are crossed by the medullary rays. Logwood has a feeble, peculiar odor, and a sweetish taste, which becomes astringent by chewing, and imparts a violet color to the saliva. It is found in the shops in the form of chips or turnings, which sometimes exhibit a shining, golden-green tint.

Lignum Guajaci.

[GUAIACUM WOOD]. Guajakholz.

[*Lignum Vitæ*]. *Pockholz.* *Franzosenholz.* *Lignum sanctum.*

Guajacum officinale *Linn.*

A heavy, dense, and hard wood, with a resinous, greenish-brown heart-wood (*duramen*), and a lighter, pale-yellow sap-wood (*alburnum*). When exposed to heat it exhales a benzoin-like odor.

The commercial raspings should not be too largely mixed with the whitish raspings of the sap-wood, or with other woods.

Lignum Quassiæ.

[QUASSIA]. Quassia.

Quassiaholz. *Lignum Quassiæ Surinamensis.*

Quassia amara *Linn.*

A light, whitish wood, having on the transverse section medullary rays, crossed by very narrow (fine) concentric rings, which are discernible by means of a lens. It occurs in cylindrical billets of about eight centimetres in thickness, covered with a thin, easily-separable bark, which is sometimes wanting. The wood has a very bitter taste.

The commercial raspings should not be employed, neither the wood of the so-called Jamaica Quassia (*Picrasma excelsa* Planchon), which occurs in pieces of the trunk, about three decimetres in thickness, having on the transverse section broader medullary rays and concentric rings, which are visible to the naked eye, and it is covered with a thicker bark.

Lignum Sassafras.

[Sassafras Wood]. Sassafras.

[*Sassafras Root*]. *Fenchelholz.*

Sassafras officinalis *Nees.*

In the form of large, branched, woody roots, consisting of crooked pieces varying in size. The root is covered with a rather thick, corky bark, externally gray and fissured, and internally of a rusty-red. The wood is light, somewhat spongy, of a pale-brownish or pale-reddish color, and on the transverse section, especially at the commencement of each annual concentric ring, it is plainly porous. It has a fennel-like odor, and a somewhat sweetish taste.

Linimentum ammoniatum.

[Liniment of Ammonia]. Flüchtiges Liniment.

[*Volatile Liniment*]. *Linimentum volatile.*

Take of Provence Olive Oil *four parts*, ... 4
Water of Ammonia *one part*. 1

Shake them together in a glass bottle until they have completely united.

It is a whitish, semi-fluid mass; the constituent parts should not separate on repose. It should be free from rancidity.

Linimentum ammoniato-camphoratum.

[Ammoniated Camphor Liniment]. Flüchtiges Kampferliniment.

[*Volatile Liniment of Camphor*].

Take of Camphorated Oil (Oleum camphoratum) *four parts*, ... 4
Water of Ammonia *one part*. 1

Shake them together in a glass bottle until they have completely united.

The Liniment is whitish, semi-fluid, and of a uniform consistence.

Linimentum saponato-ammoniatum.

[AMMONIATED SOAP LINIMENT]. Flüssiges Seifenliniment.

[*Volatile Soap Liniment*].

Take of Common Hard Soap, in shavings, *one part*. . 1
Dissolve it by digestion in
Common Water *thirty parts*, ... 30
Alcohol *ten parts*, ... 10
then add of
Water of Ammonia *fifteen parts*, ... 15
and mix.

It should be preserved in well-closed vessels.

Linimentum saponato-camphoratum.

[CAMPHORATED SOAP LINIMENT]. Opodeldok.

[*Opodeldoc*].

Take of Common Hard Soap, powdered, *sixteen parts*, . 16
Castile Soap, powdered, ... 8
Camphor, each, *eight parts*. 8
Dissolve them, with a gentle heat, in
Alcohol *three hundred and twenty parts*, . . 320
then filter the warm liquid by means of a covered funnel, and, having added,
Oil of Thyme *one part*, ... 1
Oil of Rosemary *two parts*, ... 2
Water of Ammonia *sixteen parts*, ... 16
pour it into small, wide-mouthed bottles, which should be then well closed, and allowed to cool in cold water, as quickly as possible.

The Liniment has a yellowish-white color, and a soft, semi-solid consistence. It is somewhat translucent and opalescent, melting readily with the warmth of the hand.

Linimentum saponato-camphoratum liquidum.

[SOAP LINIMENT]. Flüssiger Opodeldok.

[Liquid Opodeldoc].

Take of Castile Soap, in shavings, *thirty parts*, . . 30
Diluted Alcohol *two hundred and thirty parts*, . 230
Camphor *five parts*. 5

Dissolve with a gentle heat. Add of
Oil of Thyme *one part*, ... 1
Oil of Rosemary *two parts*, ... 2
Water of Ammonia *eight parts*.. 8

Filter the cold liquid.

It should be clear and yellowish.

Liquor Ammonii acetici.

[SOLUTION OF ACETATE OF AMMONIUM]. Essigsaure Ammoniumflüssigkeit.

[Spirit of Mindererus]. Spiritus Mindereri.

Take of Water of Ammonia *ten parts*, ... 10
add of
Diluted Acetic Acid *nine parts*, ... 9
or sufficient to effect neutralization.

Then add of
Distilled Water *a sufficient quantity*,
so that the whole shall be *thirty parts*. 30

It should be clear, colorless, entirely volatilizable, and as nearly neutral as possible. The specific gravity is from 1.028 to 1.032. It contains fifteen per cent. of acetate of ammonium. It should not become turbid on the addition of either hydrosulphuric acid, or chloride of barium.

Liquor Ammonii anisatus.

[ANISATED SPIRIT OF AMMONIA]. Anishaltige Ammoniumflüssigkeit.

Ammoniacum solutum anisatum.
Spiritus Salis ammoniaci anisatus.

Take of Oil of Anise *one part*, ... 1
dissolve it in
Alcohol *twenty-four parts*, ... 24
add of
Water of Ammonia *five parts*, ... 5
and mix.

It forms a clear and yellowish liquid.

It should be preserved in well-closed vessels.

Liquor Ammonii carbonici.

[SOLUTION OF CARBONATE OF AMMONIUM]. Kohlensaure Ammoniumflüssigkeit.

Take of Carbonate of Ammonium *one part*, . . . 1
dissolve it in
Distilled Water *five parts*. 5

A clear, colorless, completely volatilizable liquid, of a specific gravity between 1.070 and 1.074.

It should be preserved in well-closed, glass-stoppered bottles.

Liquor Ammonii carbonici pyro-oleosi.

[SOLUTION OF PYRO-CARBONATE OF AMMONIUM]. Flüssiges brenzlich-kohlensaures Ammonium.

Take of Pyro-carbonate of Ammonium *one part*, . . 1
dissolve it in
Distilled Water *five parts*, ... 5
set aside for a few days, then filter.

A clear, somewhat yellowish liquid, becoming gradually yellowish-brown; entirely volatilizable, and having a specific gravity between 1.070 and 1.074. It must be preserved in well-closed vessels, protected from the light.

Liquor Ammonii caustici.

[WATER OF AMMONIA]. Salmiakgeist.

[Solution of Ammonia. Liquor of Ammonia]. Aetzammoniakflüssigkeit. Spiritus salis ammoniaci causticus.

A transparent, colorless, and completely volatilizable liquid, without an empyreumatic odor, having the specific gravity 0.960.

It should become but slightly turbid when mixed with an equal weight of lime-water. When accurately saturated with nitric acid, and then largely diluted with distilled water, it should be rendered only slightly turbid on the addition of nitrate of silver, and should not be altered by hydrosulphate of ammonium, or hydrosulphuric acid. Oxalate of ammonium should cause no cloudiness.

It contains ten per cent. of ammonia (NH_3).

It should be preserved in well-closed glass-stoppered bottles.

Liquor Ammonii caustici spirituosus.

[SPIRIT OF AMMONIA]. Weingeistige Aetzammoniakflüssigkeit.

Spiritus Ammoniaci caustici Dzondii.

Ammoniacal gas is passed into alcohol, of the specific gravity 0.830, until the liquid shows the specific gravity of from 0.808 to 0.810.

It contains about ten per cent. of ammonia (NH_3).

When diluted with water, it behaves in the presence of reagents like water of ammonia.

It should be preserved in well-closed glass-stoppered bottles.

Liquor Ammonii succinici.

[SOLUTION OF SUCCINATE OF AMMONIUM]. Bernsteinsaure Ammoniumflüssigkeit.

Ammoniacum succinicum solutum. Liquor Cornu Cervi succinatus.

Take of Succinic Acid, powdered, *one part*, ... 1
dissolve it in
Distilled Water *eight parts*, ... 8
and add of
Pyro-carbonate of Ammonium *one part*, . . 1
or sufficient to effect neutralization.

Set the liquid aside for twenty-four hours, then filter.

A clear, brownish liquid, gradually changing to a darker brown. It has no effect on test-paper, and possesses an empyreumatic odor. Its specific gravity ranges from 1.050 to 1.054. When mixed with three times its weight of alcohol it should remain clear; and, if evaporated to dryness, it should be afterwards volatilized without a residue, at a higher temperature.

It should be preserved in well-closed vessels.

Liquor Ferri acetici.

[SOLUTION OF ACETATE OF IRON]. Essigsaure Eisenflüssigkeit.

Take of Solution of Persulphate of Iron *ten parts*, . 10
dilute it with
Distilled Water *thirty parts*, ... 30
and, while stirring, add of
Water of Ammonia *eight parts*, ... 8
previously diluted with
Distilled Water *one hundred and sixty parts*, . 160
taking care that there shall be an alkaline reaction.

The resulting precipitate is placed on a linen strainer, well washed with distilled water, then expressed until the weight shall amount to *five parts*. 5

Put this moist oxide of iron in a flask, and pour upon it
Diluted Acetic Acid *six parts*, ... 6
and set aside for several days in a cool place, stirring frequently, then filter. Add to the filtered liquid a quantity of distilled water sufficient to make the whole amount, by weight, to *ten parts*. 10

t forms a dark, reddish-brown liquid, of an acetous odor, becoming turbid by heat, and having the specific gravity of from 1.134 to 1.138, corresponding to eight per cent. of iron. When mixed with an excess of water of ammonia, the filtered liquid should not become turbid on the addition of hydrosulphuric acid; and, when evaporated to dryness, it should be afterwards volatilized, without a residue, at a higher temperature.

It should be preserved in well-closed vessels.

Liquor Ferri chlorati.

[SOLUTION OF PROTOCHLORIDE OF IRON]. Flüssiges Eisenchlorür.

Ferrum chloratum solutum. Liquor Ferri muriatici oxydulati.

Take of Pure Hydrochloric Acid *five hundred and twenty parts*. 520

Introduce it into a sufficiently large flask, and add, in small quantities at a time, of
Iron, in filings or wire, *one hundred and ten parts*. 110

When the evolution of gas has nearly ceased, place the flask in a steam-bath for several hours; then filter the liquid quickly from the undissolved iron, and mix it with

Pure Hydrochloric Acid *one part*, . . . 1

and add sufficient Distilled Water to make the whole amount, by weight, to *one thousand parts*. . . . 1000

It contains ten per cent. of iron. Its specific gravity varies from 1.226 to 1.230.

It is a clear solution, of a pale green color, and does not become turbid when mixed with alcohol. Hydrosulphuric acid should cause but a very slight white cloudiness. When mixed with an excess of solution of caustic soda, and cleared by filtration, the filtrate is not rendered turbid by hydrosulphuric acid.

It should be preserved in small, well-closed bottles.

Liquor Ferri sesquichlorati.

[Solution of Sesquichloride of Iron]. Flüssiges Eisenchlorid.

[Solution of Perchloride of Iron]. Ferrum sesquichloratum solutum. Liquor Ferri muriatici oxydati.

A clear solution of a saffron-yellowish-brown color, having a specific gravity varying from 1.480 to 1.484. It contains fifteen per cent. of iron, or forty three and a half per cent. (43.5) of anhydrous sesquichloride of iron.

When mixed with four times its volume of alcohol, and set aside for a considerable time, it should remain transparent. Diluted with water, it is not rendered turbid by chloride of barium. The diluted solution, mixed with an excess of water of ammonia, yields a filtrate, which, when supersaturated with sulphuric acid, must not decolorize a few drops of permanganate of potassium, or solution of indigo, added; nor should the filtrate be affected by hydrosulphuric acid; and, when evaporated, it is afterwards volatilized, without a residue, at a higher temperature.

It should be preserved in glass-stoppered bottles, and be protected from the light.

Liquor Ferri sulfurici oxydati.

[SOLUTION OF PERSULPHATE OF IRON]. Flüssiges schwefelsaures Eisenoxyd.

[Solution of Tersulphate of Iron].

Take of Pure Protosulphate of Iron *forty parts.* . . 40
Dissolve it in
Distilled Water *forty parts,* 40
then add of
Pure Sulphuric Acid *seven parts.* 7
Heat the mixture to the boiling point in a porcelain capsule, and very gradually add of
Pure Nitric Acid *twelve parts,* 12
or so much that, after the reaction has ceased, a small portion does no longer decolorize a solution of permanganate of potassium. Then evaporate the liquid to a resin-like mass, and dissolve it in
Distilled Water *forty parts,* 40
filter and add distilled water sufficient so that the specific gravity shall be between 1.317 and 1.319.

A clear solution, of a brownish-yellow color, and the consistence of syrup, containing eight per cent. of iron. After adding an excess of water of ammonia, the filtered liquid is not rendered turbid by hydrosulphuric acid; and, when evaporated to dryness, is afterwards volatilized, without a residue, at a higher temperature.

It should be preserved in well-closed vessels, and be protected from the light.

Liquor Hydrargyri nitrici oxydulati.

[SOLUTION OF SUBNITRATE OF MERCURY]. Flüssiges salpetersaures Quecksilberoxydul.

Hydrargyrum oxydulatum nitricum solutum. Liquor Bellostii.

Take of Subnitrate of Mercury *one hundred parts.* . . 100
Reduce it to a very fine powder in a porcelain mortar, and add of
Pure Nitric Acid *fifteen parts,* 15
dissolve, without heat, in
Distilled Water *eight hundred and eighty-five parts.* 885

A clear, colorless solution, containing ten per cent. of subnitrate of mercury. It behaves in the presence of reagents like subnitrate of mercury.

It is prepared only when wanted for dispensing.

Liquor Kali acetici.

[SOLUTION OF ACETATE OF POTASSIUM]. Flüssiges essigsaures Kali.

Kali aceticum solutum. Liquor Terræ foliatæ Tartari.

Take of Diluted Acetic Acid *one hundred parts,* . . 100
add, in small portions at a time, of
Bicarbonate of Potassium *forty-eight parts.* . 48
Heat the solution in a porcelain vessel, and add sufficient
Bicarbonate of Potassium
to effect neutralization.
Then add a sufficient quantity of
Distilled Water to make the whole amount to
one hundred and forty-two parts. 142

A clear, colorless, neutral liquid, having the specific gravity of from 1.176 to 1.180. *Three parts* should contain *one part* of dry acetate of potassium. It behaves, in the presence of reagents, like acetate of potassium.

Liquor Kali arsenicosi.

[SOLUTION OF ARSENITE OF POTASSIUM]. Fowler'sche Tropfen.

[Fowler's Solution]. Solutio arsenicalis Fowleri.

Take of Arsenious Acid, in small pieces, ... 1
Pure Carbonate of Potassium, dried, each, *one part.* 1
Place them in a test-tube, and pour upon them
Distilled Water *one part,* 1
and boil until a clear solution is obtained, then mix with
Distilled Water *about forty parts.* 40
Finally, add to the cold liquid,
Distilled Water *sufficient* so that the whole shall
be, by weight, *ninety parts.* 90
Preserve it *very cautiously*, and dispense according to legal regulations.

NOTE.—*Ninety parts* of Solution of Arsenite of Potassium contain *one part* of Arsenious Acid.

Liquor Kali carbonici.

[SOLUTION OF CARBONATE OF POTASSIUM]. Flüssiges kohlensaures Kali.

Take of Pure Carbonate of Potassium *eleven parts.* . 11
Dissolve it in
Distilled Water *twenty parts,* 20
or so much water that the specific gravity of the liquid shall be between 1.330 and 1.334. *Three parts* of the solution should contain *one part* of dry carbonate of potassium.

It should be clear and colorless. It behaves in the presence of reagents like pure carbonate of potassium.

Liquor Kali caustici.

[SOLUTION OF CAUSTIC POTASSA]. Aetzkalilauge.

[***Solution of Potassa. Liquor Potassæ***]. ***Kali hydricum solutum. Lixivium causticum.***

A clear, colorless, or slightly yellowish, very corrosive liquid, having a specific gravity of between 1.330 and 1.334; *three parts* contain *one part* of hydrate of potassium (K H O). It should effervesce but very little on addition of nitric acid. When supersaturated with diluted nitric acid, nitrate of silver should render it but slightly turbid, and chloride of barium only very slightly so.

It should be *cautiously* preserved in glass-stoppered bottles.

Liquor Natri carbolici.

[SOLUTION OF CARBOLATE OF SODIUM]. Flüssiges carbolsaures Natron.

Take of Pure Carbolic Acid *five parts.* 5
Melt it with a gentle heat, and add of
Solution of Caustic Soda *one part,* . . . 1
Distilled Water *four parts.* 4

A clear liquid of a specific gravity from 1.060 to 1.065, having a feeble alkaline reaction. Miscible with all proportions of water, and alcohol.

It is only prepared when wanted for dispensing.

Liquor Natri caustici.

[SOLUTION OF CAUSTIC SODA]. Aetznatronlauge.

[*Solution of Soda. Liquor Sodæ*]. *Natrum hydricum solutum.*

A clear, colorless or slightly yellowish, very corrosive liquid, having a specific gravity of between 1.330 and 1.334. It contains from *thirty to thirty-one per cent.* of hydrate of sodium (Na HO).

It behaves in the presence of reagents like solution of caustic potassa.

It should be *cautiously* preserved in well-closed, glass-stoppered bottles.

Liquor Natri chlorati.

[SOLUTION OF CHLORINATED SODA]. Bleichflüssigkeit.

[*Labarraque's Solution*]. *Liquor Natri hypochlorosi.*

Take of Chlorinated Lime *twenty parts*. . . . 20

Introduce it into a glass vessel, and shake it frequently with

Common Water *one hundred parts*, . . . 100

then add of

Commercial Carbonate of Sodium *twenty-five parts*, ... 25

previously dissolved in

Common Water *fifty parts*. 50

Set aside for a few hours, then decant the clear liquid.

A clear, colorless liquid, having a slight odor of chlorine. *One thousand parts* should contain at least *five parts* of active chlorine. The solution must therefore, when mixed with *forty parts* of pure protosulphate of iron, and the necessary quantity of hydrochloric acid, assume only a brown color on the addition of ferridcyanide of potassium, and must not throw down a blue precipitate.

Liquor Plumbi subacetici.

[SOLUTION OF SUBACETATE OF LEAD]. Bleiessig.

[*Goulard's Extract*]. *Acetum plumbicum s. saturninum. Plumbum hydrico-aceticum solutum.*

Take of Acetate of Lead *three parts*, ... 3
Litharge, in very fine powder, *one part*. . . 1

Mix well by rubbing them together; then introduce them into a porcelain vessel, cover it, and, by means of a steam-bath, heat the mixture until it melts into a white mass. Then add of

Warm Distilled Water *ten parts*, ... 10

stir and filter the liquid when nearly cold.

A clear, colorless liquid of a feeble alkaline reaction; having a specific gravity of between 1.235 and 1.240.

It should be *cautiously* preserved in well-closed bottles.

Liquor seriparus.

[ESSENCE OF RENNET]. Laabessenz.

[*Rennet-Wine*].

Take the fourth stomach (abomasus) of a suckling calf, wash it with water, and scrape off and collect the inner mucous membrane.

Add *three parts* of this fresh membrane . . 3
to *twenty-six parts* of Sherry Wine, ... 26
and then add of
Chloride of Sodium *one part*. 1

Macerate for three days, stir frequently, and then filter.

Essence of Rennet is a clear, yellowish liquid. It should be but slightly acidulous.

Liquor Stibii chlorati.

[SOLUTION OF CHLORIDE OF ANTIMONY]. Spiessglanzbutter.

[***Solution of Terchloride of Antimony. Muriate of Antimony. Butter of Antimony***]. ***Butyrum Antimonii s. Stibii.***

Take of Levigated Black Sulphuret of Antimony *one part*, ... 1
Hydrochloric Acid *five parts*. 5

Introduce them into a flask, and digest with a gradually augmented heat as long as gas continues to be developed. Then filter the cool liquid through asbestos, and distill from a glass retort until the distillate becomes milky when mixed with water.

Afterwards, mix the residual liquid in the retort with
Diluted Hydrochloric Acid *a quantity sufficient* so that the specific gravity shall be between 1.34 and 1.36.

Solution of Chloride of Antimony is a clear, yellowish, oily liquid. It is wholly volatilized at a moderate heat. When mixed with from four to five parts of water it forms a pulpy mass; the liquid, separated by filtration, and mixed with tartaric acid, should not become turbid on the addition of sulphate of sodium, nor blue when treated with water of ammonia.

It should be *cautiously* preserved in glass-stoppered bottles.

Lithargyrum.

[LITHARGE]. Bleiglätte.

[***Oxide of Lead***]. ***Plumbum oxydatum.***

A yellowish or reddish-yellow, heavy powder; completely soluble, or very nearly so, in diluted nitric acid, with scarcely any perceptible effervescence. This solution, when mixed with an excess of sulphuric acid, yields a filtrate, which, when supersaturated with water of ammonia, does not exhibit a blue color, and deposits but a mere trace of sesquioxide of iron. Litharge, when repeatedly boiled with diluted acetic acid, should leave only a very small amount of metallic lead behind.

It should be *cautiously* preserved.

Lithium carbonicum.

[CARBONATE OF LITHIUM]. Kohlensaures Lithion.

A white, inodorous powder, of an alkaline reaction; soluble in water and alcohol. It melts when heated, and on cooling hardens into a crystalline mass.

One part should not dissolve in less than one hundred parts of water. When dissolved in hydrochloric acid, the solution, evaporated to dryness, leaves a residue which must be completely soluble in a mixture of equal weights of alcohol and ether, and its aqueous solution must not be rendered turbid by oxalate of ammonium, or carbonate of sodium.

Lycopodium.

[LYCOPODIUM]. Bärlappsamen.

Streupulver. Semen Lycopodii.

Lycopodium clavatum *Linn.*

A very fine powder, which, when viewed under the microscope, is found to consist of very small, four-angled-roundish cells, with reticulated ridges, and having the form of a triangular pyramid, with a very convex base. Lycopodium is very mobile, adhering to the fingers, of a pale-yellow color, floating on water, with which it mixes with difficulty. When thrown into flame it burns very quickly, with a crackling noise, and without smoke.

It should be quite dry, free from foreign substances, not be mixed with the deeper colored pollen of pines, hazelnut, and other plants, all of which may be best detected by means of the microscope. Neither should it be adulterated with starch, or the flour of peas, which may be recognized by it striking a blue color with a few drops of solution of iodine. It should also be free from sand.

Macis.

[MACE]. Macis.

Muskatblüthe. Arillus Myristicæ.

Myristica fragrans *Houttuyn.*

The covering (arillus) of the fruit; it is egg-shaped, thin, somewhat horny, brittle, of an orange-yellow color, and unctuous lustre; not parted at the base, but perforated; slit at the upper part, and numerously divided. In commerce it occurs in a compressed state, or in fragments. It has a burning taste when chewed, and a peculiar aromatic odor.

Magnesia carbonica.

[CARBONATE OF MAGNESIUM]. Weisse Magnesia.

Magnesia alba. Magnesia hydrico-carbonica.

A very white, coherent mass, which is very light, devoid of taste, and readily reduced to powder. It dissolves in nitric acid with effervescence, yielding a solution which does not afford a precipitate with carbonate of ammonium, and is rendered but slightly turbid by chloride of barium, or nitrate of silver, and is not altered in the least by hydrosulphuric acid. The water in which it has been boiled, when filtered and evaporated, should leave but a very slight residue.

Magnesia citrica effervescens.

[EFFERVESCING CITRATE OF MAGNESIUM]. Brausende citronensaure Magnesia.

Take of Carbonate of Magnesium *twenty-five parts*, . 25
Citric Acid *seventy-five parts*, ... 75
Distilled Water *a sufficient quantity.*

Mix, and reduce them to a rather thick paste, which dry at a temperature not exceeding 30° C. Take of this dry mass *fourteen parts*, ... 14
and mix with
Bicarbonate of Sodium *thirteen parts*, . . . 13
Citric Acid *six parts*, ... 6
White Sugar, in very fine powder, *three parts.* 3

Moisten the mixture with a sufficient quantity of alcohol, and pass it through a tinned-iron sieve, to form a coarse, granular powder. Lastly, dry the powder in a moderately warm place.

It should be preserved in well-closed bottles.

Magnesia lactica.

[LACTATE OF MAGNESIUM]. Milchsaure Magnesia.

Take of Lactic Acid *one part*, ... 1
Distilled Water *ten parts*, ... 10
mix, heat gently, and add of
Carbonate of Magnesium *a sufficient quantity*
to effect neutralization. Then filter and evaporate, that crystals, or crystalline crusts, may form.

The salt consists of colorless, prismatic crystals, or of crystalline crusts. It is permanent in the air, and has scarcely a bitter taste. Soluble in about twenty-six parts of cold, and in three and a half parts of boiling water; insoluble in alcohol. The aqueous solution must not affect test-paper. When exposed to heat, the salt loses water, and at an increased temperature is calcined, and leaves a residue, consisting of magnesia, equal to half the weight of the salt.

Magnesia sulfurica.

[SULPHATE OF MAGNESIUM]. Bittersalz.

[*Epsom Salts*]. *Sal amarum. Sal Anglicum.*

In small, colorless, prismatic crystals, very slightly efflorescent in the air, possessing a bitter, cooling, saline taste. Soluble in three parts of cold, and in equal parts of boiling water, forming a neutral solution.

The solution is not altered by hydrosulphuric acid, or tincture of galls, nor rendered turbid by nitrate of silver. If one part of the salt, and three parts of carbonate of barium be boiled with a sufficient quantity of water, the solution, when filtered, must have no alkaline reaction.

Magnesia sulfurica sicca.

[Dried Sulphate of Magnesium]. Entwässertes Bittersalz.

Sulphate of Magnesium is allowed to fall into powder, in a moderately warm place, until it has lost one-fourth part of its weight. It is then passed through a sieve.

A fine, white powder, of the chemical purity of the crystallized salt.

It should be preserved in well-closed vessels.

When Powdered Epsom Salts (*Pulvis Magnesiæ sulfuricæ*), is prescribed, the Dried Sulphate of Magnesium (*Magnesia sulfurica sicca*), is dispensed.

Magnesia usta.

[Magnesia]. Gebrannte Magnesia.

[*Calcined Magnesia*].

A bulky, very white, and fine powder. It should dissolve in diluted sulphuric acid without effervescence. In other respects it behaves, in the presence of reagents, like carbonate of magnesium.

It should be preserved in well-closed vessels.

Manganum hyperoxydatum.

[Black Oxide of Manganese]. Braunstein.

[*Peroxide, or Binoxide of Manganese*].

In heavy crystalline, or compact masses, of a grayish-black color, and metallic lustre; they are friable, and soil the fingers. Heated with hydrochloric acid, chlorine is evolved.

When ten parts of the very finely powdered mineral is digested in two hundred parts of hydrochloric acid, with forty parts of pure protosulphate of iron, and afterwards heated to the boiling point, a liquid is formed, which, when filtered, must not assume a blue color on the addition of ferridcyanide of potassium. It must, therefore, contain no less than sixty per cent. of pure peroxide of manganese.

Manna.

[Manna]. Manna.

Fraxinus Ornus *Linn.*

The purest Manna [Flake Manna], consists of pieces from seven to twenty centimetres in length, and from two to four centimetres in width, being more or less flattened, cannulated, or triangular. They are dry, light, friable, and only slightly viscid, having a white or yellowish-white color, and a fibrous fracture. Their taste is sweet, without being acrid. This Manna is dispensed when Select or Cannulated Manna (*Manna electa vel canellata*), is prescribed.

Common Manna [Manna in sorts], or Gerace Manna, occurs in masses, and is composed of agglutinated fragments or grains, of a whitish or brownish color. They are somewhat viscid, and have a sweet and subnauseous, acrid taste.

The coarse, fat or Puglia Manna (*Manna crassa, pinguis seu de Puglia*), in crumbling, soft, viscid, and brownish masses, mixed with a great deal of impurities, and often in a state of fermentation, should be rejected.

Mastix.

[Mastic]. Mastix.

[*Mastich*]. *Mastiche. Resina Mastiche.*

Pistacia Lentiscus *Linn.* γ. **Chia** *DC.*

In somewhat spherical, pale-yellow, friable tears, of about the size of a pea, externally dusty. The freshly-broken pieces are glassy, shining and transparent. Mastic becomes soft when chewed. It dissolves partially in cold and in boiling alcohol.

Mel.

[Honey]. Honig.

Apis mellifica *Linn.*

When freshly collected, honey is a translucent, syrupy liquid. By keeping, it is changed into a granular, opaque mass, of a whitish-yellow, yellow, or brownish-yellow color. It has a very sweet taste, and a peculiar odor, and forms, with water and with diluted alcohol, a slightly turbid solution.

Honey must be free from acidity, and not be adulterated with flour.

Mel depuratum.

[CLARIFIED HONEY]. Gereinigter Honig.

Take of Honey *one part*, ... 1
Common Water *two parts*. 2

Heat them in a tinned vessel, and let them stand at a temperature of about 100° C. for an hour, avoiding ebullition. Filter the liquid when it has cooled to between 50° and 40° C., and evaporate, by means of a steam-bath, to the consistence of a syrup, and lastly strain.

Clarified honey is clear, and forms a clear mixture with water. It has a yellowish-brown color, and should be free from sour or empyreumatic odor and taste.

It should be preserved in a cool place.

Mel rosatum.

[HONEY OF ROSE]. Rosenhonig.

Take of Pale Rose *one part*, ... 1
Hot Water *six parts*. 6

Set aside for a night, then express and filter. Mix the filtered liquid with
Clarified Honey *ten parts*, ... 10
and evaporate to the consistence of a syrup, by means of a steam-bath, and strain.

Honey of Rose is clear, with a brown color.

It should be preserved in a cool place.

Minium.

[RED LEAD]. Mennige.

[*Red Oxide of Lead*].

A heavy, orange-red powder. Partially soluble in nitric acid, leaving the brown peroxide of lead; but completely soluble, or nearly so, in the same acid on the addition of oxalic acid or sugar. The solution thus produced, treated with an excess of sulphuric acid, and filtered, must contain no copper, and but a mere trace of iron.

Mixtura gummosa.

[GUM ARABIC MIXTURE]. Gummi-Mixtur.

Take of Gum Arabic, in very fine powder, ... 15
White Sugar, in very fine powder, each, *fifteen parts*, ... 15
Dissolve them in
Distilled Water *one hundred and seventy parts*. 170
It is prepared only when wanted for dispensing.

Mixtura oleoso-balsamica.

[HOFFMAN'S BALSAM OF LIFE]. Hoffmann'scher Lebensbalsam.

Balsamum Vitæ Hoffmanni.

Take of Oil of Lavender, ... 1
Oil of Cloves, ... 1
Oil of Cinnamon (cassia), ... 1
Oil of Thyme, ... 1
Oil of Lemon, ... 1
Oil of Mace, ... 1
Oil of Orange flowers, each, *one part*, . . 1
Balsam of Peru *three parts*, ... 3
Alcohol *two hundred and forty parts*. . . 240

Mix and set aside for several days in a cool place, shake occasionally, and filter.

A clear, brownish-yellow liquid.

It should be preserved in well-closed vessels.

Mixtura sulfurica acida.

[SULPHURIC ACID MIXTURE]. Haller'sches Sauer.

In place of Elixir acidum Halleri. [***Haller's Acid Elixir***].

Take of Pure Sulphuric Acid *one part*, ... 1
and add, by drops, while stirring, to
Alcohol *three parts*. 3

A clear, colorless liquid of the specific gravity from 0.998 to 1.002.

It should be preserved in glass-stoppered bottles.

Mixtura vulneraria acida.

[THEDEN'S VULNERARY WATER]. Theden'sches Wundwasser.

Take of Vinegar *six parts*, ... 6
Diluted Alcohol *three parts*, ... 3
Diluted Sulphuric Acid *one part*, . . . 1
Clarified Honey *two parts*. 2

Mix and filter.

It is clear and yellow at first; afterwards it becomes brownish.

Morphinum.

[MORPHIA]. Morphin.

In white, shining, prismatic crystals, not efflorescent in the air; or in a crystalline powder. It has an alkaline reaction and a bitter taste. It is scarcely dissolved by cold water, ether or benzole; but it is more readily soluble in alcohol, and freely so in diluted acids, solutions of caustic potassa, and soda, and also in lime-water. When gradually heated, morphia fuses, and, at an elevated temperature, chars and burns without leaving a residue. It is dissolved, without coloration, by sulphuric acid; but, if afterwards heated and allowed to cool, a blood-red color is produced in the mixture by a very little nitric acid.

It should be *cautiously* preserved.

Morphinum aceticum.

[ACETATE OF MORPHIA]. Essigsaures Morphin.

A white or whitish powder, having a slight odor of acetic acid and a very bitter taste. Soluble in about twenty-four parts of water, to which has been added a few drops of diluted acetic acid. It dissolves with greater difficulty in alcohol.

It behaves in the presence of reagents like morphia.

It should be *cautiously* preserved in closed vessels.

Morphinum hydrochloricum.

[MURIATE OF MORPHIA]. Salzsaures Morphin.

[***Hydrochlorate of Morphia***].

In white crystals of a silky lustre, frequently united in tufts; of a very bitter taste. Soluble in twenty parts of cold water, and in sixty parts of alcohol; both solutions are neutral.

It behaves in the presence of reagents like morphia.

Preserve it *cautiously*.

Morphinum sulfuricum.

[SULPHATE OF MORPHIA]. Schwefelsaures Morphin.

In colorless, light, acicular crystals of a silky lustre; readily soluble in water and in alcohol, forming neutral solutions.

It behaves in the presence of reagents like morphia.

Preserve it *cautiously*.

Moschus.

[MUSK]. Moschus.

Moschus moschiferus ***Linn.***

Musk is at first in the form of an unctuous mass, but afterwards crumbles into grains of various sizes, with a brown color and fatty lustre. If triturated it may be spread out in a thin layer. It is secreted in a peculiar sac, lined internally with a thin, brown membrane, from which the musk is removed for use, and separated from adhering membranes and hairs. The taste is bitterish, and the odor peculiar, very persistent, and exceedingly penetrating. The sacs are almost semi-globular in form, from three to four centimetres in width, somewhat flattened on one side, and without hairs; on the other side convex, with yellowish-brown, appressed hairs (stiff and of a darker shade at the apex), disposed in a concentric manner around the two orifices near the middle of the sacs.

Care should be taken against adulterated musk: where the sacs have been opened and the genuine musk partially removed, and afterwards filled with foreign substances. Russian or Kabardine musk should be entirely rejected; the sacs of which are filled with a paler mass, of a much weaker and urinous odor.

Mucilago Cydoniæ.

[MUCILAGE OF QUINCE SEED]. Quittenschleim.

Take of Quince Seed *one part*, ... 1
Rose Water *fifty parts*. 50

Let them stand for half an hour, shaking frequently, then strain.

Mucilago Gummi Arabici.

[MUCILAGE OF GUM ARABIC]. Gummischleim.

Take of Gum Arabic *one part*, ... 1
wash it with distilled water, then dissolve it in
Distilled Water *two parts*, ... 2
and strain.

Mucilago Salep.

[MUCILAGE OF SALEP]. Salepschleim.

Take of Powdered Salep *one part*, ... 1
Cold Common Water *ten parts*. 10
Shake them well together in a flask, and add of
Boiling Common Water *ninety parts*, . . . 90
and shake again, until cold.

It should be freshly prepared for dispensing.

Myrrha.

[MYRRH]. Myrrhe.

Gummi-resina Myrrha.

Balsamodendron Ehrenbergianum *Berg,* perhaps also
Balsamodendron Myrrha *Nees.*

Myrrh occurs in pieces of irregular forms and variable sizes, covered with a fine powder or dust. The pieces are uneven on the surface, sometimes roundish in shape; have a yellowish or reddish-brown color, are friable, and, when broken, the fractured surface presents a waxy lustre, and a paler or deep reddish-brown color, and is sometimes marked with light colored veins. Myrrh has a peculiar balsamic odor and a bitter taste. Of a given quantity, the larger part is dissolved by water, forming a yellowish-brown and turbid solution, but only the lesser part is taken up by alcohol, yielding a reddish-yellow solution, which assumes a violet color on the addition of nitric acid.

Dark-brown pieces of a disagreeable odor, the alcoholic solution of which is not colored violet by nitric acid, or pieces which are entirely soluble, or merely swell up in water, are to be rejected.

Natrium chloratum purum.

[PURE CHLORIDE OF SODIUM]. Reines Kochsalz.

[***Common or Culinary Salt. Muriate of Soda***]. ***Natrum Muriaticum purum.***

In small, white, cubic crystals, or in crystalline grains, of a salty taste; soluble in two and eight-tenths parts of water. When heated it decrepitates.

An aqueous solution is neutral, and is not rendered turbid by hydrosulphuric acid, hydrosulphate of ammonium, oxalate of ammonium, nitrate of barium, or carbonate of sodium.

Natrum aceticum.

[ACETATE OF SODIUM]. Essigsaures Natron.

Terra foliata Tartari crystallisata.

In prismatic, colorless, inodorous and transparent crystals; efflorescent in the air; soluble in three parts of cold, and in equal parts of boiling water; also soluble in alcohol. When heated they first undergo the watery fusion, then become anhydrous and enter into igneous fusion, and finally, at a red-heat, are decomposed, emitting the odor of acetone.

When dissolved in about forty parts of water, the solution must not become turbid on the addition of hydrosulphuric acid, chloride of barium, or nitrate of silver.

Natrum bicarbonicum.

[BICARBONATE OF SODIUM]. Doppelkohlensaures Natron.

In very white, inodorous, concrete, crystalline crusts or pieces, permanent in the air, having a mild saline and slightly alkaline taste. Soluble in fourteen parts of cold water, but insoluble in alcohol. A solution of the salt in one hundred parts of water, is not altered by hydrosulphuric acid. When supersaturated with nitric acid, chloride of barium and nitrate of silver cause but a slight cloudiness in the solution. If six grammes of an aqueous liquid containing three decigrammes of corrosive chloride of mercury be mixed with a solution of two grammes of the bicarbonate of sodium in thirty grammes of cold water, the mixture must become but slightly cloudy after three minutes' repose.

Natrum carbonicum crudum.

[COMMERCIAL CARBONATE OF SODIUM]. Rohes krystallisirtes kohlensaures Natron.

[*Sal Soda*]. *Soda. Natrum carbonicum crystallisatum crudum. Sal Sodæ crudus.*

In large, colorless crystals, or in crystalline masses, containing from thirty-three to thirty-five per cent. of anhydrous carbonate of sodium. The aqueous solution, supersaturated with nitric acid, should be rendered but very slightly turbid by chloride of barium or nitrate of silver. Neither the alkaline solution, nor one acidulated with hydrochloric acid, should be affected by hydrosulphuric acid.

Natrum carbonicum purum.

[Pure Crystallized Carbonate of Sodium]. Reines krystallisirtes kohlensaures Natron.

Natrum carbonicum depuratum. Sal Sodæ depuratus.

In colorless, transparent crystals, of an alkaline taste, efflorescent in the air, soluble in two parts of cold, and in one-fourth part of boiling water; forming alkaline solutions.

Neither the alkaline solution, nor one acidulated with hydrochloric acid, should be altered by hydrosulphuric acid. A solution, supersaturated by nitric acid, should not be rendered turbid by nitrate of silver or nitrate of barium.

It should be preserved in well-closed vessels.

Natrum carbonicum siccum.

[Dried Carbonate of Sodium]. Getrocknete Soda.

Coarsely powdered, pure crystallized Carbonate of Sodium is allowed to effloresce in a warm place until it has lost about half its weight. The dried, white powder is then passed through a sieve and preserved in a well-closed vessel.

This dried soda is dispensed when Powdered Carbonate of Sodium is prescribed.

Natrum nitricum.

[Nitrate of Sodium]. Gereinigter Chilisalpeter.

[***Cubic Nitre. Chili Saltpetre***]. ***Nitrum cubicum.***

In colorless, transparent, rhomboidal crystals. They are anhydrous, permanent in dry air, and have a cooling, saline, somewhat bitter taste. Soluble in two parts of cold, and in less than its own weight of boiling water.

An aqueous solution should not become turbid on the addition of hydrosulphuric acid, or carbonate of sodium; and nitrate of barium, or nitrate of silver should render it but very slightly cloudy. The solution, shaken with bisulphide of carbon, which has been mixed with chlorine water, must not communicate a brownish-yellow or violet-red color to the former. Neither must bisulphide of carbon, when shaken with the watery solution, to which has been added diluted sulphuric acid, and a little zinc, assume a violet-red color.

Natrum phosphoricum.

[PHOSPHATE OF SODIUM]. Phosphorsaures Natron.

In colorless, transparent, oblique-rhomboidal crystals, efflorescent in dry air. It has a mild saline taste, and is soluble in six parts of cold, and in two parts of boiling water, with an alkaline reaction. It should not effervesce with any of the acids.

The aqueous solution, acidulated with a little nitric acid, should become but very slightly turbid with chloride of barium, and nitrate of silver. Neither should the alkaline solution, nor one acidulated with hydrochloric acid, be affected by hydrosulphuric acid.

It should be preserved in well-closed vessels.

Natrum pyrophosphoricum.

[PYROPHOSPHATE OF SODIUM]. Pyrophosphorsaures Natron.

In colorless, oblique-rhombic prisms, permanent in the air. When heated they lose water, at an increased temperature undergo the watery fusion, and on cooling form a transparent, crystalline mass. When dissolved in ten parts of cold water, the solution has an alkaline reaction, and yields, on the addition of nitrate of silver, a white precipitate, the liquid at the same time becomes neutral.

The aqueous solution, acidulated with nitric acid, should become but very slightly turbid with chloride of barium, or nitrate of silver. Hydrosulphuric acid does not change the alkaline, or the acidulated solution.

Natrum pyrophosphoricum ferratum.

[Ferro-pyrophosphate of Sodium]. Pyrophosphorsaures Eisenoxyd-Natron.

Take of Pyrophosphate of Sodium *two hundred parts*. . 200
Rub to powder, and, avoiding heat, pour upon it
Cold Distilled Water *four hundred parts*. . . 400
While stirring constantly, add, in successive small portions, of
Solution of Sesquichloride of Iron *eighty-one parts*, ... 81
previously diluted with
Distilled Water *two hundred and twenty parts*, . 220
with the precaution, that a new portion of the liquid is added only after each previously formed precipitate has been redissolved.

The greenish liquid obtained in this manner is filtered, and mixed with
Alcohol *one thousand parts*. 1000

The resulting precipitate is washed with a little alcohol, expressed between folds of bibulous paper, and dried at a gentle heat.

It forms a white, amorphous powder, dissolving slowly in cold water, forming a greenish liquid, which yields a precipitate on the addition of alcohol.

The solution is decomposed when boiled, while yielding a white precipitate.

It should be preserved in well-closed vessels.

Natrum Santonicum.

[Santonate of Sodium]. Santoninsaures Natron.

In colorless, transparent, tabular, or laminar crystals, of a bitter, saline taste, and alkaline reaction. Soluble in three parts of cold water, and in twelve parts of alcohol, but it dissolves much more readily in boiling water, and boiling alcohol. The aqueous solution deposits santonine on the addition of acids. An alcoholic solution of potassa colors it red. Light scarcely affects the salts.

It should be *cautiously* preserved.

Natrum subsulfurosum.

[HYPOSULPHITE OF SODIUM]. Unterschwefligsaures Natron.

Natrum hyposulfurosum.

In colorless, transparent, inodorous prisms, permanent in the air, having a saline, afterwards bitterish taste. They readily dissolve in water, forming a feebly alkaline solution.

If hydrochloric acid be added to an aqueous solution, it becomes turbid after a while, and disengages sulphurous acid. A strong aqueous solution yields, with chloride of barium, a white precipitate, which must be entirely soluble in a larger quantity of water.

A solution of one part of the salt with two parts of water, should dissolve, at least, one part of iodine, which solution must be colorless, and should not change the color of test-paper.

It should be preserved in well-closed vessels.

Natrum sulfuricum.

[SULPHATE OF SODIUM]. Glaubersalz.

*[**Glauber's Salt**]. **Natrum sulphuricum depuratum. Sal mirabile Glauberi depuratum.***

In colorless, transparent crystals, which readily effloresce in the air, and deliquesce when exposed to heat; soluble in three parts of cold water, in a third part of water at a temperature of 33° C., and in two-fifths at a temperature of 100° C., forming a solution which should not affect test-paper.

An aqueous solution is not altered by hydrosulphuric acid, or hydrosulphate of ammonium; and nitrate of silver should cause but a very slight cloudiness.

Natrum sulfuricum siccum.

[DRIED SULPHATE OF SODIUM]. Entwässertes Glaubersalz.

It is prepared from Crystallized Sulphate of Sodium, like Dried Carbonate of Sodium (Natrum carbonicum siccum).

It should be preserved in a well-closed vessel.

This preparation is dispensed when Powdered Sulphate of Sodium is prescribed.

Olea ætherea.

[ESSENTIAL OILS]. Aetherische Oele.

[*Distilled Oils. Volatile Oils*].

The essential oils are mostly prepared by distillation, more rarely by expression.

They should be clear, and possess the odor of the substances from which they are prepared in a high degree. They must entirely volatilize by heat, and mix with all proportions of the fixed oils, and absolute alcohol, forming clear solutions. They are so slightly soluble in water, that if shaken with a large bulk of it, the essential oils scarcely suffer diminution of volume. Most of the essential oils are lighter than water.

They should be preserved in well-closed vessels, in a cool place, and be protected from the light.

Oleum Amygdalarum.

[EXPRESSED OIL OF ALMOND]. Mandelöl.

[*Almond Oil*].

It is prepared from Sweet or Bitter Almonds. The seeds are coarsely powdered, inclosed in a bag, and expressed between cold plates. The cake is then powdered, and the expression repeated as before. The oil is set aside for a while, then filtered.

It should be clear. It has a yellowish color, and a peculiar, mild odor, without rancidity. It does not thicken in the cold.

It should be preserved in well-closed vessels.

Oleum animale æthereum.

[ETHEREAL ANIMAL OIL]. Aetherisches Thieröl.

[*Rectified Animal Oil. Dippel's Animal Oil*]. *Oleum animale Dippelii.*

Crude animal oil (oleum animale fœtidum) is distilled with a gentle heat, by means of a sand-bath, as long as a thin oil passes over, which is to be mixed with *four times its weight* of water, and redistilled as long as the distillate continues to be colorless, or but slightly yellow. The oil is afterwards separated from the water.

The oil is transparent, colorless, or slightly yellow, and possesses a very strong odor. Oil that has acquired a brown color should be rejected.

It should be preserved in small, well-closed bottles, which should be kept under water.

Oleum Anisi.

[OIL OF ANISE]. Anisöl.

A thin, colorless, or slightly yellow, oil. It concretes between 6° and 18° C., and forms a crystalline mass. It is soluble in from four to five parts of alcohol.

Oleum Aurantii Corticis.

[OIL OF ORANGE]. Pomeranzenschalenöl.

A thin, yellowish oil, which, with five parts of alcohol, forms a turbid solution.

Oleum Aurantii Florum.

[OIL OF ORANGE FLOWERS]. Pomeranzenblüthenöl.

[*Oil of Neroli*]. *Oleum Florum Naphæ. Oleum Neroli.*

A thin, yellowish, or reddish-yellow oil, soluble in an equal weight of alcohol.

Oleum Bergamottæ.

[OIL OF BERGAMOT]. Bergamottöl.

Citrus Bergamia *Risso.*

A thin, pale yellow, or greenish-yellow oil, soluble in all proportions of alcohol.

Oleum Cacao.

[BUTTER OF CACAO]. Kakaobutter.

[*Oil of Theobroma. U. S. P.*] *Butyrum Cacao.*

Theobroma Cacao *Linn.*

It is yellowish-white, of a feeble peculiar odor, and bland taste. It is of a firmer consistency than mutton suet, and melts at a temperature of 30° C.

Oleum Cajeputi.

[Oil of Cajeput]. Cajaputöl.

Melaleuca Leucadendron ***Linn.*****, et Melaleuca minor** ***Smith.***

A green or yellowish-green oil, soluble in all proportions of alcohol.

Oil contaminated with copper should be rejected.

Oleum Cajeputi rectificatum.

[Refined Oil of Cajeput]. Gereinigtes Cajaputöl.

Take of Oil of Cajeput *one part*, ... 1
Common Water *six parts*. 6

Distill as long as a colorless, or slightly yellow oil passes over.

Oleum Calami.

[Oil of Calamus]. Kalmusöl.

A yellow, or brownish-yellow, thickish oil, soluble in all proportions of alcohol.

Oleum Camphoratum.

[Camphorated Oil]. Kampferöl.

[*Liniment of Camphor*].

Take of Camphor *one part*. 1
Dissolve it in
Provence Olive Oil *nine parts*. 9

It should be preserved in well-closed vessels.

Oleum Carvi.

[OIL OF CARAWAY]. Kümmelöl.

A thin, colorless, or pale-yellowish oil, soluble in all proportions of alcohol.

Oleum Caryophyllorum.

[OIL OF CLOVES]. Nelkenöl.

A thickish, yellowish, or yellowish-brown oil, heavier than water, soluble in all proportions of alcohol.

Oleum Chamomillæ æthereum.

[OIL OF GERMAN CHAMOMILE]. Aetherisches Kamillenöl.

A thick, dark-blue oil, having at a low temperature nearly the consistence of butter; soluble in from eight to ten parts of alcohol.

Oleum Chamomillæ infusum.

[INFUSED OIL OF CHAMOMILE]. Fettes Kamillenöl.

In place of Oleum Chamomillæ coctum.

Take of German Chamomile *two parts*, ... 2
Alcohol *one part*. 1

Mix, and set aside in a well-closed vessel for several hours, then, having added of
Provence Olive Oil *twenty parts*, ... 20
digest in a steam-bath, shaking occasionally, until the alcohol is all evaporated, then express, set aside for a few days, and filter.

It is clear, and of a yellowish-green color.

Oleum Cinnamomi Cassiæ.

[OIL OF CINNAMON]. Zimmtöl.

[*Oil of Cassia*]. *Zimmtkassienöl. Oleum Cinnamomi.*

Oleum Cassiæ.

A thickish, yellowish, or yellowish-brown oil, heavier than water, soluble in all proportions of alcohol.

Oleum Cinnamomi Zeylanici.

[OIL OF CEYLON CINNAMON]. Zeylonisches Zimmtöl.

A thickish, yellowish, or brownish-red oil, heavier than water, soluble in all proportions of alcohol.

Oleum Citri.

[OIL OF LEMON]. Citronenöl.

Oleum de Cedro.

A thin oil; when recently prepared somewhat cloudy, becoming clear and yellowish by age, and dissolving in from ten to twenty parts of alcohol.

Oleum Cocois.

[COCO-NUT OIL]. Kokosöl.

[*Cocoa-nut Oil*].

Cocos nucifera *Linn.*

A white, fatty substance, solid and somewhat granular when cold, becoming soft at 15° C., and liquid at 23° C., having a peculiar odor.

Oleum Crotonis.

[CROTON OIL]. Krotonöl.

Tiglium officinale *Klotzsch.*

A thickish, yellowish, or brownish-yellow fixed oil. The taste is at first bland, but becomes very acrid on the tongue, and produces blisters. It has a disagreeable odor. It is soluble in thirty-six parts of alcohol, and easily soluble in ether.

It should be *cautiously* preserved.

Oleum Fœniculi.

[OIL OF FENNEL]. Fenchelöl.

A thin, colorless or yellowish oil, congealing between a temperature of 4° and 18° C., to a crystalline mass, soluble in from one to two parts of alcohol.

Oleum Hyoscyami infusum.

[INFUSED OIL OF HYOSCYAMUS]. Fettes Bilsenkrautöl.

In place of Oleum Hyoscyami coctum.

It is prepared from Hyoscyamus Leaves, like Oleum Chamomillæ infusum.

It has a brownish-green color.

Oleum Jecoris Aselli.

[COD-LIVER OIL]. Leberthran.

Gadus Morrhua *Linn.*, Gadus Callarias *Linn.*,

Gadus Carbonarius *Linn.*, and of other species of Gadus.

A clear, yellowish or reddish-brown oil, of a fishy odor, without rancidity.

Oleum Juniperi.

[OIL OF JUNIPER BERRIES]. Wachholderbeeröl.

Oleum Fructuum Juniperi.

A thin, colorless, or slightly yellowish oil, soluble in twelve parts of alcohol, forming a turbid solution.

Oleum Juniperi empyreumaticum.

[OIL OF CADE]. Kadeöl.

Oleum cadinum.

Juniperus Oxycedrus ***Linn.***

An empyreumatic, dark-brown semi-fluid oil, similar to tar.

Oleum Lauri.

[OIL OF BAYS]. Lorbeeröl.

[***Expressed Oil of Bays***]. ***Oleum laurinum. Oleum Lauri unguinosum s. expressum.***

A granular, green, or yellowish-green oil, of the consistence of an ointment, having the aromatic odor of the bay-berries; soluble in one and a half parts of ether.

The green color is not changed by water of ammonia.

Oleum Lavandulæ.

[OIL OF LAVENDER]. Lavendelöl.

A thin, yellowish, or greenish-yellow oil, soluble in its own weight of alcohol.

Oleum Lini.

[FLAXSEED OIL]. Leinöl.

[Linseed Oil].

A clear, yellowish, fixed, drying oil, of a bland taste, and a peculiar odor. It concretes at a temperature of 16° C. Soluble in one and a half parts of ether, and in five parts of absolute alcohol.

Oleum Lini sulfuratum.

[SULPHURATED FLAXSEED OIL]. Geschwefeltes Leinöl.

[Balsam of Sulphur]. Balsamum Sulphuris.

Take of Flaxseed Oil *six parts*. 6

Heat it in a sufficiently capacious iron vessel, and add of

Sublimed Sulphur *one part*. 1

Boil them, stirring constantly with a spatula, and avoiding the boiling over of the mixture, until they have united into a homogeneous mass.

It has the consistence of [European] turpentine, and a reddish-brown color. It is completely soluble in oil of turpentine.

Oleum Macidis.

[OIL OF MACE]. Macisöl.

Muskatblüthenöl.

A thin, colorless, or yellowish oil, soluble in six parts of alcohol.

Oleum Majoranæ.

[OIL OF SWEET MARJORAM]. Meiranöl.

A thin, yellowish oil, soluble in all proportions of alcohol.

Oleum Menthæ crispæ.

[OIL OF CURLED-MINT]. Krauseminzöl.

A thin oil, becoming thicker, and pale-yellow or greenish by age. Soluble in all proportions of alcohol.

Oleum Menthæ piperitæ.

[OIL OF PEPPERMINT]. Pfefferminzöl.

A thin, colorless oil, sometimes of a yellowish or greenish color, becoming thicker by age. Soluble in equal parts of alcohol.

Oleum Myristicæ.

[EXPRESSED OIL OF NUTMEG]. Muskatnussöl.

[Butter of Nutmegs]. Muskatbutter. Oleum Nucistæ expressum. Butyrum Nucistæ.

An oil of the consistence of suet, occurring in commerce in quadrangular cakes, of an orange-yellow color, with a yellowish-white, or reddish-mottled appearance, having the peculiar odor of the nutmeg. It is completely soluble in four parts of boiling ether, and melts between 45° and 48° C.

Oleum Olivarum.

[OLIVE OIL]. Olivenöl.

[Sweet Oil].

There are two kinds in use:

1. Best Olive Oil, or Provence Olive Oil (*Oleum Olivarum optimum seu Provinciale*), of a pale-yellow color, a feeble, peculiar odor, and a bland taste.

2. Common or Green Olive Oil (*Oleum Olivarum commune seu viride*), of a yellow or greenish-yellow color, and a more or less disagreeable odor. Both oils congeal into an unctuous, granular mass at a temperature of a few degrees above 0° C.

Oleum Papaveris.

[POPPY OIL]. Mohnöl.

A yellowish, fixed, drying oil, almost without odor, having a bland taste.

Oleum Petræ Italicum.

[CRUDE PETROLEUM]. Steinöl.

Petroleum crudum.

A clear, yellowish or reddish liquid, iridescent, having a peculiar bituminous odor; soluble in the fixed and essential oils, also in ether and absolute alcohol. It dissolves with difficulty in alcohol. Specific gravity from 0.75 to 0.85.

Oleum phosphoratum.

[PHOSPHORATED OIL]. Phosphorhaltiges Oel.

Take of Phosphorus, well dried, *one part*, . . . 1
Expressed Oil of Almonds *eighty parts*. . . 80

Having introduced them into a flask, place it in hot water to melt the phosphorus. Then shake the vessel, and, when the solution is completed, set aside, in a cool place, for half an hour. Pour off cautiously the cold oil from the, perchance, slight deposit of phosphorus.

It is clear, fuming, having the odor of phosphorus.

It is only prepared when wanted for dispensing.

Oleum Ricini.

[CASTOR OIL]. Ricinusöl.

Oleum Castoris vel Palmæ Christi.

Ricinus communis *Linn.*

A rather thick fixed oil, colorless or yellowish, congealing by cold, and having a bland taste. Soluble in all proportions of alcohol.

Rancid Castor Oil, and that which is acrid and irritating to the throat, should be rejected.

Oleum Rosæ.

[OIL OF ROSE]. Rosenöl.

Otto or Attar of Roses.

Rosa moschata *Miller*; Rosa Damascena *Miller*, and of other species of Rose.

A pale-yellow, volatile oil, rather thick and crystalline, liquefying between 15° and 25° C. Soluble at 17° C. in ninety parts of alcohol.

Oleum Rosmarini.

[OIL OF ROSEMARY]. Rosmarinöl.

Oleum Anthos.

A thin, colorless oil, soluble in equal parts of alcohol.

Oleum Sabinæ.

[OIL OF SAVINE]. Sadebaumöl.

A thin, yellowish oil, soluble in equal parts of alcohol.
It should be *cautiously* preserved.

Oleum Sinapis.

[OIL OF MUSTARD]. Aetherisches Senföl.

[*Volatile Oil of Mustard. Essential Oil of Mustard*].

A thin, yellowish, or yellow oil, heavier than water, of a very pungent odor. It is soluble in fifty parts of water, and in all proportions of alcohol.

When the oil is shaken with three times its volume of pure sulphuric acid, keeping the mixture cool while shaking, it should, after twelve hours, be converted into a thick or crystalline mass, which should not have a brown color.

Preserve it *cautiously* in well-closed vessels.

Oleum Succini rectificatum.

[RECTIFIED OIL OF AMBER]. Gereinigtes Bernsteinöl.

A thin, colorless, or yellowish oil, soluble in from ten to twelve parts of alcohol.

Oleum Terebinthinæ.

[OIL OF TURPENTINE]. Terpenthinöl.

[Spirits of Turpentine]. Spiritus Terebinthinæ.

A thin, colorless, or slightly yellowish oil. An oil having an empyreumatic odor should be rejected.

Oleum Terebinthinæ rectificatum.

[RECTIFIED OIL OF TURPENTINE]. Gereinigtes Terpenthinöl.

It is prepared from Oil of Turpentine, like Rectified Oil of Cajeput.

It is thin, colorless, and soluble in about twelve parts of alcohol.

Oleum Terebinthinæ sulfuratum.

[SULPHURATED OIL OF TURPENTINE]. Schwefelbalsam.

Balsamum Sulphuris terebinthinatum.

Take of Sulphurated Flaxseed Oil *one part*, . . . 1
Oil of Turpentine *three parts*. 3

Dissolve by digestion. After repose decant the clear liquid from the deposit.

It is clear, and of a reddish-brown color.

Oleum Thymi.

[OIL OF THYME]. Thymianöl.

A thin, colorless, sometimes yellowish or greenish oil, soluble in equal parts of alcohol.

Oleum Valerianæ.

[OIL OF VALERIAN]. Baldrianöl.

A somewhat thick, brownish, or greenish-yellow oil, soluble in all proportions of alcohol.

Olibanum.

[OLIBANUM]. Weihrauch.

[*Frankincense*]. *Gummi-resina Olibanum. Thus.*

Boswellia papyrifera *Hochstetter.*

In roundish tears of different sizes, having a whitish, brownish-yellow or a brownish-red color, with a powdery surface. The tears are friable, have a waxy lustre; when chewed they soften and dissolve to some extent, producing a sensation of coldness in the mouth. They melt partially by heat, and diffuse a balsamic odor. Alcohol dissolves the greater part, and, when they are triturated with water, a milky fluid is formed.

Opium.

[OPIUM]. Opium.

Mohnsaft. Laudanum. Meconium.

Papaver somniferum *Linn.*

Opium occurs generally in roundish or somewhat flattened lumps, having a weight of about three-fourths of a kilogramme. They are enveloped in poppy leaves, and covered with the fruits of a species of Rumex. The masses are somewhat soft when fresh, internally of a pale-brown color, consisting of grains or small tears, which are visible on the cut surface. Opium is darker when dry, and has a reddish-brown, shining fracture. It is partially soluble in alcohol and in water, and has a nauseous, narcotic odor, and a bitter taste.

Dried and powdered opium should contain no less than ten per cent. of morphia.

It should be *cautiously* preserved.

Oxymel Colchici.

[OXYMEL OF COLCHICUM]. Herbstzeitlosen-Sauerhonig.

Take of Vinegar of Colchicum *one part*, ... 1
Clarified Honey *two parts*. 2

Mix, evaporate in a steam-bath to *two parts*, . . 2
and strain.

It is clear with a brownish-yellow color.

It should be preserved in a cool place.

Oxymel Scillæ.

[OXYMEL OF SQUILL]. Meerzwiebel-Sauerhonig.

It is prepared from Vinegar of Squill like Oxymel of Colchicum.

It is clear, with a yellowish-brown color.

It should be preserved in a cool place.

Oxymel simplex.

[SIMPLE OXYMEL]. Sauerhonig.

Take of Diluted Acetic Acid *one part*, ... 1
Clarified Honey *forty parts*. 40

Mix them.

It is clear, with a yellowish-brown color.

Pasta Guarana.

[GUARANA]. Guarana.

[*Paullinia*].

Paullinia sorbilis ***Martius.***

Guarana generally occurs in the form of cylindrical rolls, less frequently in flattened or globular masses. They are prepared by removing the seeds from the pods, drying them in the sun, powdering, and, with a little water, kneading them into a paste, which is dried in the sun, or by the smoke of a fire. The masses are hard, and have a dark-brown color, a peculiar odor, and an astringent, bitterish taste, which is similar to that of cacao. They break generally with a flat surface, which has a feeble lustre; not unfrequently containing separate seeds, and they dissolve partially in water.

Pasta gummosa.

[MARSHMALLOW PASTE]. Gummipasta.

[Opaque Gum Paste]. Pasta Althææ.

Take of Gum Arabic, ... 200
White Sugar, each, *two hundred parts.* . . . 200
Dissolve them in
Cold Distilled Water *six hundred parts.* . . . 600
Allow the liquid to settle, strain from the impurities, and evaporate it in a copper kettle, placed in a steam-bath, to the consistence of honey, while stirring with a wooden spatula. Then add of
Fresh White of Eggs *one hundred and fifty parts,* 150
previously beaten to a thick froth. Continue the stirring, while evaporating the paste with a gentle heat, until it drops with some difficulty from the spatula in motion. Finally, having added
Oleosaccharate of Neroli* *one part,* 1
pour the mass into paper capsules, and dry it in a warm place. Then remove from the capsules, and cut it into strips, and preserve it in a dry place.
Marshmallow Paste is very white.

Pasta Liquiritiæ.

[LIQUORICE PASTE]. Süssholzpasta.

Pasta Glycyrrhizæ.

Take of Liquorice Root, cut, *one part.* 1
Pour upon it
Distilled Water *twenty parts,* 20
macerate for twelve hours, then strain and filter, and, having diluted the liquid with
Distilled Water *ten parts,* 10
add, and dissolve
Gum Arabic, previously washed with water, *fifteen parts,* 15
White Sugar *nine parts.* 9

---

* See Elæosacchara, page 67.

Pour the liquid through a woolen strainer, heat it for an hour in a steam-bath, and, having removed the film, evaporate immediately, without stirring, until a drop placed on a cold metal plate congeals to the consistence of stiff jelly. Then, after removing the film, pour the mass into paper capsules, which have been placed inside tin ones. Dry the paste sufficiently with a gentle heat, remove it from the paper capsules with the aid of steam, cut it into narrow strips, and dry it properly.

The paste has a brownish-yellow color, is translucent, and free from empyreuma.

It should be preserved in well-closed vessels, in a dry place.

Phosphorus.

[PHOSPHORUS]. Phosphor.

A translucent, white or yellowish, wax-like substance, which occurs generally in the form of small cylindrical sticks. When exposed to the air it diffuses an odor somewhat similar to garlic. It is luminous in the dark; ignites very readily, and melts under water at a temperature of 44° C., to a clear, oily fluid. It is insoluble in water, slightly soluble in alcohol and ether, more readily so in the fixed and essential oils, and dissolves with still greater facility in bisulphide of carbon. It contains frequently traces of sulphur and arsenic.

It should be *very cautiously* preserved under water, in a glass bottle which must be inclosed in a tin case.

Pilulæ aloëticæ ferratæ.

[FERRATED PILLS OF ALOES]. Italienische Pillen.

[***Italian Pills***]. ***Pilulæ Italicæ nigræ.***

Take of Pure Dried Protosulphate of Iron,
Aloes, powdered, each, *equal parts.*

Mix, and beat them into a pilular mass by means of a sufficient quantity of alcohol, and divide into pills, each weighing ten centigrammes.

They have a shining, black color.

Pilulæ Ferri carbonici.

[PILL OF CARBONATE OF IRON]. Vallet'sche Pillen.

[Vallet's Mass]. Pilulæ ferratæ Valleti.

Take of Pure Protosulphate of Iron *twenty-four parts,* 24
and dissolve it in boiled Distilled Water *seventy-five parts,* to which has been added *one-twentieth part* of its weight of Simple Syrup.

Likewise dissolve
Pure Carbonate of Sodium *twenty-five parts,* . 25
in *seventy parts* of Distilled Water, sweetened as above, and filter.

Mix the liquids in a vessel, which should be completely filled by them, and close it tightly. Pour off the supernatant liquid from the precipitate, and fill the vessel again with sweetened water. Shake well and let it stand for twelve hours. Then pour off the liquid again from the precipitate, and repeat the operation with sweetened water, until only a mere trace of sulphate and carbonate of sodium may be detected. Then inclose the precipitate in a linen cloth saturated with simple syrup, express forcibly, and mix, without delay, with
Honey *fourteen parts,* 14
previously warmed by means of a steam-bath.

Evaporate the mass in the steam-bath until the residue shall be *twenty-one parts,* 21
so that a pilular mass may be formed, which should contain one-half its weight of carbonate of protoxide of iron.

Twenty-five decigrammes of the mass, after the necessary addition of powdered marshmallow root, are formed into twenty-five pills which are dusted with powdered cassia. Each pill contains five centigrammes (0.05) of carbonate of iron.

Pilulæ Jalapæ.

[PILLS OF JALAP]. Jalapenpillen.

Take of Jalap Soap *three parts,* 3
Jalap Root, powdered, *one part.* 1

Beat them into a pilular mass, and divide into pills, each weighing *ten centigrammes,* and dust them with lycopodium.

Pilulæ odontalgicæ.

[ODONTALGIC PILLS]. Zahnpillen.

[Tooth-ache Pills].

Take of Opium, powdered, ... 5
Belladonna Root, powdered, ... 5
Pellitory Root, powdered, each, *five grammes*, . 5
Yellow Wax *seven grammes*, ... 7
Expressed Oil of Almonds *two grammes*, . . 2
Oil of Cajeput,
Oil of Cloves, each, *fifteen drops*.

Mix them in a moderately warm mortar, and beat into a pilular mass; form it into pills, each weighing five centigrammes, and dust them with powdered cloves. They are of a soft consistence.

They should be preserved in a well-closed vessel.

Pix liquida.

[TAR]. Theer.

Resina empyreumatica liquida.

A thick, oily, blackish-brown, semi-translucent liquid, heavier than water. It has an unpleasant empyreumatic smell, and a bitter, burning taste.

Warm water, shaken with tar, acquires an acid reaction.

It is procured by the destructive distillation of the wood of the Abies genus, or of Beech.

Pix navalis.

[BLACK PITCH]. Schiffspech.

Pix nigra. Pix solida. Resina empyreumatica solida.

A black, opaque, resinous mass, brittle when cold, becoming soft between the fingers by the warmth of the hand, and having the odor of tar, from which it has been procured by distilling off the volatile portion.

Placentæ Seminis Lini.

[FLAXSEED OIL-CAKE]. Leinkuchen.

[*Linseed Oil-cake*].

The cake left after the expression of linseed oil.

Plumbum aceticum.

[ACETATE OF LEAD]. Essigsaures Bleioxyd.

[*Sugar of Lead*]. *Bleizucker. Saccharum Saturni depuratum.*

In colorless, translucent crystals, soluble in two parts of cold, and in half its weight of boiling water, also in eight parts of alcohol.

The aqueous solution throws down a white precipitate on the addition of water of ammonia; the liquid separated from the precipitate by filtration should have no blue color.

It should be preserved *cautiously* in well-closed vessels.

Plumbum Iodatum.

[IODIDE OF LEAD]. Jodblei.

An orange-yellow powder, soluble in one thousand and three hundred parts of cold, and in two hundred parts of boiling water, leaving no residue, and forming a colorless solution. It is fused and decomposed by heat, emitting violet-colored vapors.

It should be *cautiously* preserved.

Plumbum tannicum pultiforme.

[Soft Tannate of Lead]. Breiartiges gerbsaures Bleioxyd.

Cataplasma ad decubitum.

Take of Oak Bark, cut, *eight parts*. 8
Boil it for half an hour in
Common Water *a sufficient quantity* to yield *forty parts*, ... 40
of strained decoction.
To the filtered decoction, add, while stirring, of
Solution of Subacetate of Lead *about four parts*, 4
or add as long as a precipitate is thrown down.

The precipitate, collected on a filter, consists of about *three parts*, by weight, and is of the consistence of a rather thick liniment. Mix this precipitate, in a gallipot, with
Alcohol *one part*. 1

It is prepared only when wanted for dispensing.

Potio Riveri.

[Solution of Citrate of Sodium]. River'scher Trank.

[River's Effervescing Draught].

Take of Citric Acid *four parts*, ... 4
Distilled Water *one hundred and ninety parts*. . 190
Introduce them into a bottle, which should be nearly filled, dissolve by agitation, and add gradually of
Pure Crystallized Carbonate of Sodium *nine* parts. 9

As soon as it is dissolved by agitation, close the bottle.
It is prepared only when wanted for dispensing.

Pulpa Tamarindorum cruda.

[Crude Tamarind Pulp]. Rohes Tamarindenmus.

[*Tamarind*]. *Tamarindi.* *Fructus Tamarindorum.*

Tamarindus Indica *Linn.*

The pods of the East India Tamarind afford, after the removal of the external cortical shell (exocarp), and bruised, a fleshy, tough, brownish-black pulp, containing the papery membranes of the cells, and bundles of fibres, and also the hard, chestnut-brown seeds. Tamarind pulp has a vinous odor, and an agreeable, acid, and feeble astringent taste.

Egyptian Tamarind pulp should be rejected. It consists of black, hard, lenticular masses, about fifteen centimetres wide, as also the pulp, which has been mixed with tartaric acid, and often made with water, into a soft, black mass; frequently mouldy, and of a very sour taste. The soft, yellowish-brown pulp of West India Tamarind, frequently in a state of fermentation, should also be rejected.

A piece of bright iron, left in contact with the pulp for some time, should not exhibit a deposit of copper.

Pulpa Tamarinda depurata.

[Prepared Tamarind Pulp]. Gereinigtes Tamarindenmus.

Mix equal parts of Crude Tamarind Pulp, and Hot Water, and set them aside, stirring frequently, until the mass assumes a uniform consistence.

Then pass the pulp through a hair-sieve, by means of a wooden spatula, and evaporate it in a porcelain vessel, with a steam-bath, to the consistence of thick extract.

Afterwards, mix with each *six parts*, ... 6
of the pulp, while still warm,
White Sugar, powdered, *one part*. 1

It has a blackish-brown color, and an agreeable sour taste. It should be preserved in a cool and dry place. Care should be taken that it is not contaminated with copper, which may be detected with a polished iron blade.

Pulvis aërophorus.

[EFFERVESCING POWDER]. Brausepulver.

Take of Bicarbonate of Sodium *ten parts*, . . . 10
Tartaric Acid *nine parts*, ... 9
White Sugar *nineteen parts*. 19

Convert each ingredient separately into very fine powder, then dry, and mix them.

The powder should be preserved in well-closed vessels, or be prepared when called for.

It should be quite dry, and effervesce strongly when thrown into water.

Pulvis aërophorus Anglicus.

[SODA POWDERS]. Englisches Brausepulver.

Soda-Powder.

Take of Bicarbonate of Sodium, powdered, *two grammes*. 2
Dispense it in blue or red paper.
Take of Tartaric Acid *one and a half grammes*. . . 1½
Dispense it in white paper.

Pulvis aërophorus laxans.

[APERIENT EFFERVESCING POWDERS]. Abführendes Brausepulver.

[***Seidlitz Powders***]. ***Seidlitzpulver. Pulvis aërophorus Seidlitzensis.***

Take of Tartrate of Potassium and Sodium, powdered, *seven and a half grammes*, ... 7½
Bicarbonate of Sodium, powdered, *two and a half grammes*. 2½

Mix them.

Dispense separately with the above
Tartaric Acid, powdered, *two grammes*. . . 2

REMARK.—This formula is intended for one dose.

Pulvis aromaticus.

[AROMATIC POWDER]. Aromatisches Pulver.

Take of Cassia Bark, powdered, *five parts*, ... 5
Small Cardamoms, powdered, *three parts*, . 3
Ginger, powdered, *two parts*. 2
Mix intimately.

Pulvis arsenicalis Cosmi.

[ARSENICAL POWDER OF CÔME]. Cosmisches Pulver.

Take of Red Sulphuret of Mercury *one hundred and twenty parts*, ... 120
Animal Charcoal *eight parts*, ... 8
Dragon's Blood *twelve parts*, ... 12
Arsenious Acid *forty parts*. 40

Mix intimately, so as to form a powder.
It should be *very cautiously* preserved.

Pulvis gummosus.

[COMPOUND POWDER OF GUM ARABIC]. Gummipulver.

Take of Gum Arabic, powdered, *three parts*, ... 3
Liquorice Root, powdered, *two parts*, . . 2
White Sugar, powdered, *one part*. . . . 1
Mix them.

Pulvis Ipecacuanhæ opiatus.

[COMPOUND POWDER OF IPECACUANHA]. Dower'sches Pulver.

[Dover's Powder]. Pulvis Doweri.

Take of Sulphate of Potassium, powdered, *eight parts*, . 8
Opium, powdered, ... 1
Ipecacuanha, powdered, each, *one part*. . . 1

Mix them intimately together.
It should be *cautiously* preserved in well-closed vessels.
REMARK.—*Ten parts* contain *one part* of opium.

Pulvis ad Limonadam.

[LEMONADE POWDER]. Limonadenpulver.

Pulvis refrigerans Ph. Badensis.

Take of White Sugar, powdered, *one hundred and twenty grammes*, ... 120
Citric Acid, powdered, *ten grammes*, . . 10
Oil of Lemon *one drop*.
Mix them intimately together.
The powder is only prepared when wanted for dispensing.

Pulvis Liquiritiæ compositus.

[PECTORAL POWDER]. Brustpulver.

Pulvis Glycyrrhizæ compositus. Pulvis pectoralis Kurellæ.

Take of Senna, powdered, ... 2
Liquorice Root, powdered, each, *two parts*, . 2
Fennel Seed, powdered, ... 1
Washed Sulphur, each, *one part*, . . . 1
White Sugar, powdered, *six parts*. . . . 6
Mix them.

Pulvis Magnesiæ cum Rheo.

[MAGNESIA AND RHUBARB]. Kinderpulver.

[***Infant Powder***]. ***Pulvis infantum. Pulvis antacidus.***

Take of Carbonate of Magnesium *sixty parts*, . . 60
Oleosaccharate of Fennel* *forty parts*, . . 40
Rhubarb, powdered, *fifteen parts*. . . . 15
Mix them.
It should be preserved in well-closed vessels.

---

* See Elæosacchara, page 67.

Pulvis temperans.

[Refrigerant Powder]. Niederschlagendes Pulver.

Pulvis refrigerans Ph. Germaniæ.

Take of	Nitrate of Potassium, powdered, *one part*, .	1
	Bitartrate of Potassium, powdered, *three parts*,	3
	White Sugar, powdered, *six parts*. . . .	6

Mix them.

Radix Alkannæ.

[Alkanet Root]. Alkannawurzel.

Alkanna tinctoria *Tausch.*

The root is subcylindrical, nearly simple, with numerous heads (crowns), and about one and a half centimetres in thickness. It has a dark purple, soft, light bark, which readily separates in laminæ, and imparts a red color to the saliva, and a purple color to alcohol, the fixed and some essential oils, and the cerates, but not to water. The ligneous portion is hard, whitish, and is often fissured radially.

The drug, when consisting principally of the bark, is to be preferred; the root destitute of the bark should be rejected.

Radix Althææ.

[Marshmallow Root]. Altheewurzel.

Eibischwurzel.

Althæa officinalis *Linn.*

The root is long, about the thickness of a finger, white when deprived of its outer bark. The liber is rather thick, strongly fibrous and flexible. The ligneous portion is fleshy; brittle and farinaceous when dry. It has a somewhat sweet, and very mucilaginous taste.

The root of the plant, either growing wild or cultivated, may be taken up in the beginning of the spring, or in autumn, and should be separated from the root-stock, woody and decayed parts, deprived of the outer cortical portion, and quickly dried.

Radix Angelicæ.

[GARDEN-ANGELICA ROOT]. Engelwurzel.

Radix Archangelicæ.

Archangelica officinalis ***Hoffmann.***

The roots are long, from four to six millimetres in thickness, soft, furrowed, issuing from a rather thick, upright root-stock (caudex), which is about eight centimetres in length, somewhat spongy, and exhibiting close, slightly elevated rings towards the upper part. The bark of the root is rather thick, of a grayish-brown color externally, white within, and provided with numerous yellow, shining receptacles, filled with balsamic matter, the vessels being much broader than their pores. The ligneous portion is yellowish, and radially marked. The root produces a burning sensation in the mouth when chewed, with a sweetish taste at first, afterwards bitter. It has a strong odor.

Worm-eaten roots should be rejected. The root of *Angelica silvestris* Linn., must not be substituted; it is smaller, thinner, having fewer and much smaller balsamic receptacles.

The root of the second year's growth should be gathered in the spring, and should be well dried, and preserved in well-closed vessels.

Radix Arnicæ.

[ARNICA ROOT]. Arnikawurzel.

Wohlverleihwurzel.

Arnica montana ***Linn.***

The root-stock (rhizome) is horizontal or oblique, varying in length; about three millimetres in thickness. It is hard, contorted, premorse (ending abruptly), having obscure rings, a rough, brown surface, and being furnished with rootlets. Its bark is rather thick, white within, surrounding with its balsamic ducts the yellowish, radially marked, ligneous portion, which is provided with a large and whitish pith. The rootlets are rather long, and about one millimetre in thickness, hard, brittle; externally brown, whitish internally, and their bark is provided with balsamic ducts.

The root, when chewed, causes an acrid, burning sensation in the mouth; has a bitterish taste, and a strong, peculiar odor.

The root is to be collected in the spring or autumn, and should not be confounded with the roots of *Achyrophorus maculatus*, *Hieracia*, *Betonica* and *Fragaria*, in which the balsamic ducts are wanting; neither with the roots of *Virgaurea* and *Eupatorium*, which have a thicker root-stock.

Radix Artemisiæ.

[MUGWORT ROOT]. Beifusswurzel.

Artemisia vulgaris *Linn.*

The roots are rather long, about two millimetres in thickness, contorted, somewhat branched and furrowed; their color is externally of a light-brown, and white within; issuing from all sides of a perpendicular, cylindrical, woody root-stock, which is about two and a half centimetres in thickness. The transverse section of the roots exhibits an interrupted ring of brownish-red balsamic ducts, arranged around the central ligneous portion.

The roots should be gathered in the spring or autumn, separated from the root-stock, and from the decayed portion, but should not be washed. They are to be dried immediately, and preserved in a well-closed vessel, and be renewed once a year. In preparing the powder from the recently dried roots, the central ligneous portion should be rejected.

The powder should also be preserved in well-closed vessels.

Radix Asari.

[ASARABACCA]. Haselwurzel.

Rhizoma Asari.

Asarum Europæum *Linn.*

The root-stock is obtusely-quadrangular, elongated, about two millimetres in thickness, remotely jointed, somewhat dichotomously branched; branches single-jointed. It has a grayish-brown color. A dark-brown ring divides the thickish bark from the radiated, thin, brownish, ligneous portion, which incloses a large, farinaceous pith. The taste, when chewed, is burning and pepper-like. The odor is camphorous.

Before dispensing, the root should be separated from both the kidney-shaped, petiolated leaves, which generally remain attached to the commercial drug.

Radix Bardanæ.

[Burdock Root]. Klettenwurzel.

Lappa officinalis *Allione*, and of other species of Lappa.

The root is nearly simple, long, as thick as a finger, wrinkled, and of a grayish-brown color externally, pale-brown internally. It has a thickish bark, which is furnished frequently, within, with minute, tomentose, lacunal, whitish cavities. The ligneous portion is radiated, inclosing a thin, lacerated, snow-white pith. The root, when chewed, is mucilaginous and sweetish, afterwards somewhat bitter. Its odor is rather feeble.

The root of the first year's growth should be gathered in autumn, and that of the second year's in spring, and should be preserved in a dry place. It occurs generally cut lengthwise.

Radix Belladonnæ.

[Belladonna Root]. Belladonnawurzel.

Atropa Belladonna *Linn.*

The root is long, about four centimetres thick, provided with long simple branches; fleshy when fresh, and farinaceous when dry; longitudinally striped and wrinkled, and of a yellowish-gray color externally, and whitish internally; provided with closely-situated, yellowish, porous, woody bundles (fascicles), which are more scattered toward the centre, and are arranged in a circle around the root. It has a powdery fracture.

The root may be gathered, either in the spring or autumn, from the not too old, wild-growing plant, but it must not be scraped. The root occurs frequently sliced lengthwise. Roots that are woody, tough, dark-colored, mouldy, or worm-eaten, should be rejected.

It should be *cautiously* preserved, and not kept longer than a year.

Radix Carlinæ.

[CARLINE THISTLE]. Eberwurzel.

Carlina acaulis *Linn.*

The root is long, about two and a half centimetres thick, nearly simple, and often many-headed; furrowed longitudinally, and of a brown color externally; very frequently split lengthwise to the centre, and the woody portion laid open, which is netted-wavy, and internally of a rather pale color. The somewhat thin bark, and the fleshy wood, are radiated and furnished with brownish-red resiniferous ducts. The root has a burning, bitter taste, and a disagreeable odor.

It should be collected in the autumn.

Radix Colombo.

[COLUMBO]. Kolombowurzel.

[*Calumba Root*]. *Radix Columbo.*

Jateorrhiza Calumba *Miers*, (**Cocculus palmatus** *Wallich*).

In nearly circular segments, three to four centimetres in diameter, and from four to twelve millimetres in thickness, wrinkled and grayish-brown externally; farinaceous, and of a greenish- or brownish-yellow color internally. The segments are concave on both sides, inside of the broad elevated margins, or raised again around the centre. A dark-colored ring, traversed by numerous radial lines, divides the raised margin. From the concave surfaces emerge scattered woody bundles (fascicles). The root has a very mucilaginous, and a very bitter taste. It is colored blue when sprinkled with solution of iodine.

Radix Gentianæ.

[GENTIAN ROOT]. Enzianwurzel.

Gentiana lutea *Linn.*

A very long, somewhat branched root, two and a half centimetres or more in thickness; the heads (crowns) are short and numerous. The root occurs generally split longitudinally; the pieces are furrowed lengthwise, and marked with close, transverse wrinkles at the upper portion. Externally the root is yellowish, or reddish-brown, and internally it is of a reddish, or orange-brown color. It is brittle when dry, often spongy and porous, and has an uneven fracture. The cortical portion is thin, and separated from the thick, fleshy, ligneous portion by a dark-colored ring. It has a very bitter, persistent taste. The root of other species of Gentian, about as thick as a finger, rigid, externally more of a grayish-brown color, but otherwise very similar to the genuine root, need not be rejected; but care must be taken against the admixture of the root of White Hellebore (*Veratrum*).

The root should be gathered in the spring.

Radix Helenii.

[ELECAMPANE]. Alantwurzel.

Radix Enulæ.

Inula Helenium *Linn.*

It occurs in commerce in long slices of the main root, about four centimetres in breadth, together with the cylindrical, thinner, decorticated branches, sometimes also split longitudinally; of a yellowish, or brownish-white color. It has a bitter taste, and a peculiar odor. The dried root is hard and brittle, but is tough when moist. It is furnished internally with numerous small, shining oil-receptacles. The somewhat thick bark is separated by a dark-colored ring from the fleshy, ligneous portion, which contains narrow, lemon-yellow, fascicled vessels, and broad medullary rays. The pith in the main root is rather broad (large), but it is wanting in the branches.

The root may be gathered either in the spring or autumn.

Radix Hellebori viridis.

[EUROPEAN GREEN HELLEBORE]. Grüne Nieswurzel.

Helleborus viridis *Linn.*

The rhizome (root-stock) is closely beset with rootlets, and is branched towards the top. The branches are ascending, nearly spindle-shaped, annulated, and about four centimetres long, and four millimetres thick, showing on a transverse section, a rather thick bark, and a somewhat large pith, with broad, inwardly-truncated bundles of woody fibres (fascicles), which are somewhat separated, and arranged in an interrupted ring. The rootlets are close together, about ten centimetres long, and one and a half millimetres in thickness. They are brittle, externally, as well as the rhizome, brownish-black, and internally mostly of a dirty-white.

The root should not be confounded with the root of *Helleborus niger* L., *Adonis vernalis* L., *Actæa spicata* L. The pedate, herbaceous, unequally and sharply-serrated leaves, remaining attached to the rhizome, should be removed before dispensing. The root of *Helleborus niger* is characterized by the branches of the root-stock exhibiting, on a transverse section, narrow, wedge-shaped bundles of woody fibres, and by being furnished with rootlets of a foot in length, and about three millimetres in thickness, and having a dark-brown color: the root of *Adonis* by a nearly simple and almost conical rhizome, beset very closely all around with rootlets. The root of *Actæa* is known by its spreading-branched rhizome, and long, tough rootlets.

The root should be gathered in early spring, before the plant begins to blossom, or in the autumn.

It should be *cautiously* preserved.

Radix Ipecacuanhæ.

[IPECACUANHA]. Brechwurzel.

Cephaëlis Ipecacuanha *Willdenow.*

The root is contorted, from two to four millimetres in thickness, tapering towards both ends. It has a knotty appearance in consequence of incomplete, puffed, closely-situated rings. The cortical portion is thick, horny; externally varying in color from a dark to a light-brown; internally brownish, without radial marks, and easily separable from the whitish, thin, ligneous portion.

It should be *cautiously* preserved.

In preparing the powder, the ligneous portion, constituting about one-fourth the weight of the root, must be rejected.

Radix Levistici.

[LOVAGE ROOT]. Liebstöckelwurzel.

Levisticum officinale ***Koch.***

A rather long root, about four centimetres in thickness. It is soft, slightly branched; externally marked with transverse wrinkles; furrowed longitudinally, and of a yellowish-brown color; internally of a pale-yellow color. The cortical portion is rather thick, lacunose, and provided with orange-colored balsamic ducts, which are arranged in a scattered, nearly concentric manner. The ligneous portion is dense and soft. Its odor is peculiar, and its taste disagreeably sweetish and burning.

Radix Liquiritiæ glabræ.

[LIQUORICE ROOT]. Spanisches Süssholz.

[***Spanish Liquorice Root***]. ***Radix Glycyrrhizæ Hispanica.***

Glycyrrhiza glabra ***Linn.***

A very long, nearly simple root, about two centimetres in thickness. It is heavy, externally of a brownish-gray color, and longitudinally furrowed; internally of a deep-yellow color. The bark is rather thick, the inner portion of which, as well as the hard, coarsely and rigidly-fibrous, dense wood, is marked on the transverse section with linear, medullary rays.

The root has a sweet, and slightly acrid taste.

Spanish Liquorice Root should not be used for the preparation of powder; for that purpose only the Decorticated Root (*Radix Liquiritiæ mundata*), should be selected.

Radix Liquiritiæ mundata.

[DECORTICATED OR PEELED LIQUORICE ROOT]. Süssholzwurzel.

[***Russian Liquorice Root***]. ***Radix Liquiritiæ Russica. Radix Glycyrrhizæ echinatæ.***

Glycyrrhiza echinata ***Linn.***

A long root, about four centimetres in thickness, being decorticated, and mostly separated from the large root-stock (corm). It has a yellow color. The liber is rather thin; the ligneous portion is thick, light, fissured radially, and has a very fibrous fracture. It has a very sweet taste.

Radix Ononidis.

[Rest-harrow Root]. Hauhechelwurzel.

Ononis spinosa *Linn.*

A very long, tough and flexible root, about as thick as a finger, deeply furrowed longitudinally; many-headed; heads frequently rather long. The cortical portion is very thin, and externally of a deep-brown color. The ligneous portion is hard, whitish, and fibrous; the transverse section shows eccentric, rather plain, irregular, fan-like rays. It has a sweetish-bitter and burning taste.

The root may be gathered either in the spring or autumn. It occurs in commerce generally in longitudinal slices.

Radix Pimpinella.

[Burnet Saxifrage and Great Pimpinel]. Pimpinell-wurzel.

Pimpinella Saxifraga et Pimpinella magna *Linn.*

A rather long root, often many-headed, from the thickness of a quill to that of the little finger, mostly simple and straight. It is furrowed longitudinally, warty, and at the upper part marked with transverse wrinkles. It has a brown-yellowish color. The cortical portion is thick, and internally either snow-white or yellowish. When snow-white, it is traversed by narrow, yellowish rays, containing small, brownish-red, resiniferous ducts; when yellowish, the transverse section exhibits brownish rays, which are confluent around the lemon-yellow, radiated, woody portion, forming a brown ring. The root has a sweet but hot taste when chewed, and a hircine odor.

The roots should be gathered in the beginning of spring, or in the latter part of autumn, from the plants designated above.

The root of the black variety of Burnet Saxifrage (*Pimpinella Saxifraga varietas nigra*), may also be employed. It is externally black, or brownish-black, and the bark internally is marked with gray or bluish rays. But it must not be confounded with the root of Mountain Parsley (*Peucedanum Oreoselinum* Moench), the ligneous portion of which consists of an interrupted woody ring, composed of numerous wedge-shaped, vascular bundles, arranged in a radial manner; nor with the root of Cow-parsnip or Bear's-claw (*Heracleum Sphondylium* L.), which is paler, more spongy, and lacunose, and furnished with fewer resiniferous ducts, and frequently consists of strong, branched, uneven crowns (rhizomes), beset with rootlets.

Radix Pyrethri.

[PELLITORY ROOT]. Bertramwurzel.

Radix Pyrethri Germanica.

Anacyclus officinarum ***Hayne.***

A long, simple, brittle root, about four millimetres in thickness, externally grayish-brown, and wrinkled longitudinally; internally of a lighter shade. The bark is rather thick, furnished with a ring of balsamic ducts, and the woody portion presents a radiated structure. When chewed, the root has a burning taste, and causes a copious flow of saliva.

The root must be separated, before dispensing, from the adherent branches and leaves. The root of Italian Pellitory (*Pyrethrum Italicum*), about the thickness of a finger, and which is often deteriorated by age, and worm-eaten, should be rejected.

Radix Ratanhæ.

[RHATANY ROOT]. Ratanhawurzel.

Krameria triandra ***Ruiz et Pavon.***

A woody root, with a rather thick trunk, many-headed at the top, and branched below. The branches are long, about one and a half centimetres thick, cylindrical, divaricate, and sometimes occur without the main trunk. The bark is thin, cinnamon-colored, and has a slightly fibrous fracture, and a very astringent, bitterish taste; the woody portion is somewhat paler, almost tasteless, very finely radiated, porous, and at least six times thicker than the bark.

The Rhatany brought from Peru, in its entire state, and not that which is partly decorticated, should alone be employed. The root imported from Grenada, or from Texas and Brazil, all of which have a thicker bark, should be rejected.

Radix Rhei.

[RHUBARB]. Rhabarber.

Undetermined species of Chinese Rhubarb.

Consisting of pieces (segments) of various forms; hard, completely peeled or trimmed, frequently perforated, breaking with an uneven surface, externally yellow, and generally covered with a powder. They are internally marbled, with alternating white and red lines, radiately disposed, but variously winding, and intersecting each other. The root is gritty between the teeth when chewed, and imparts a yellow color to the saliva. It has a peculiar odor and taste. The dark-brown, spongy, worm-eaten, and mouldy rhubarb, should be rejected.

The root is imported from China, either overland, by way of Moscow, and is then called Russian, or Moscow Rhubarb; or by sea, *via* Canton, and is then known as Chinese, or East India Rhubarb.

The Russian drug—formerly very highly prized, but not so much valued at present—is distinguished from the Chinese by its darker color, lighter weight, and by the very numerous whitish and red figures, radially arranged on the transverse section.

The following kinds of Rhubarb, cultivated in Europe, should not be employed: that which is known as Austrian Rhubarb, presenting on the cross section alternating red and white radial lines, which are straight; and the so-called English Rhubarb, which is furnished, only towards the circumference, with distinct radial lines, and is marked towards the centre with white and red spots, being without radial figures.

Powdered Rhubarb should be preserved in well-closed vessels.

Radix Saponariæ.

[SOAPWORT]. Seifenwurzel.

Saponaria officinalis ***Linn.***

The root is rather long, terete, gradually tapering, about the thickness of a goose-quill and upwards, wrinkled lengthwise, and furnished with the remains of a stem, which is provided with protuberant nodes. The bark is externally brownish-red, internally white, and separated by a dark-colored ring from the ligneous portion, which is not radiated, of a pale lemon-yellow color, whitish and medullary in the middle.

The root is acrid when chewed, producing a foam in the mouth, and has at first a sweetish taste, afterwards somewhat bitter.

The root may be gathered in the spring or autumn.

Radix Sarsaparillæ.

[SARSAPARILLA]. Sassaparille.

Radix Sassaparillæ vel Salsaparillæ.

Smilax medica *Schlechtendal*, and of other species of Smilax.

The roots are very long, about six millimetres in thickness, striped externally, and of a grayish-brown or brownish-red color, consisting of a middle bark (*mesophlœum*), which is solid, rather thick, either mealy and white, or horny and brownish; of a closed woody ring, and a white mealy pith; not furnished with complete medullary rays. The corm (rhizome), from which the secondary roots spring, frequently accompanies them in the commercial drug, but should be separated before dispensing.

The Mexican Sarsaparilla, which is deeply furrowed, and has a shriveled and thin middle bark, and a rather thick woody body, should be rejected, as well as all the lacerated, lean, or such as have a strawy appearance.

Radix Scammoniæ.

[SCAMMONY ROOT]. Scammoniawurzel.

Convolvulus Scammonia *Linn.*

A very long, cylindrical, often many-headed root, about two centimetres in thickness, longitudinally ribbed, and of a brown color externally; paler within, and furnished with resinous specks. The bark is thin, and the woody portion consists, as shown on a cross section, of scattered but close porous woody parts, radially arranged, and separated by the cellular tissue.

It should not be confounded with Turpeth Root (*Convolvulus Turpethum*), which exhibits, on a cross section, separated woody cylinders, of various thicknesses, around the radiated porous wood, inside the thick bark.

Radix Senegæ.

[SENEKA ROOT]. Senegawurzel.

Polygala Senega *Linn.*

A subcylindrical root, tuberculous at the top (*basis*), about six millimetres in thickness, gradually tapering towards the lower extremity; somewhat branched and twisted; provided with a sharp, keel-shaped process on the concave side of the root, but is knobby on the other side. It has a yellowish or grayish-brown color. The cortical portion is rather thick, yellowish within. The woody part is yellow, and, on the opposite side to the one keeled, it is flat or concave. The root has a feeble odor, and when chewed produces an acrid sensation in the fauces.

Radix Serpentariæ.

[SERPENTARIA]. Virginische Schlangenwurzel.

[*Virginia Snakeroot*].

Aristolochia Serpentaria *Linn.*

It consists of a horizontal, contorted, somewhat flattened root-stock (rhizome), two to three millimetres in thickness, furnished along the upper side with the short and thin remnants of the stems, on the lower side with numerous very thin, brittle, pale-brown rootlets, about eight centimetres in length. The woody portion of the rhizome is thicker on the lower than on the upper side, and unequally radiated. The wood of the rootlets is four- or five-angled. Serpentaria has a bitter taste, and when rubbed a camphorous odor.

It should be preserved in well-closed vessels.

Radix Taraxaci.

[DANDELION ROOT]. Löwenzahnwurzel.

Taraxacum officinale *Weber.*

The dried root; about thirty centimetres in length, and at the top (*basis*) about two and a half centimetres in thickness. It is cylindrical, tapering gradually toward the lower extremity; generally with numerous heads, and not much branched. It is furrowed longitudinally, and has externally almost a blackish-brown color. The bark is thick; white internally, and spongy; presenting on the transverse section numerous concentric rings. The woody portion is porous, and of a lemon-yellow color. It has a bitter taste.

The root should be collected in the autumn.

Radix Taraxaci cum herba.

[ROOT AND HERB OF DANDELION]. Löwenzahnwurzel mit dem Kraute.

The fresh plant, gathered in the spring; it gives out a milky juice when wounded. The root is somewhat fleshy, of a more or less pale or blackish-brown color externally. The leaves are arranged in the form of a rosette (rosulate); they are runcinate, denticulate, nearly smooth. It has a sweetish-bitter taste.

It is used for the preparation of extract.

Radix Valerianæ.

[VALERIAN ROOT]. Baldrian.

Radix Valerianæ minoris vel montanæ.

Valeriana officinalis *Linn.*

The root-stock (corm), about four centimetres long, and two and a half centimetres thick—sometimes provided with stolons—is beset all around with very numerous, long, terete, striated rootlets, about two millimetres in thickness, white when fresh, and grayish-brown when dried. Their cortical portion is brownish within, and the woody part is thin, and of a somewhat lighter shade. Valerian is acrid, and bitter when chewed, and has a strong, peculiar odor.

It should be gathered in the autumn, dried, and preserved in closed vessels.

Resina Draconis.

[DRAGON'S BLOOD]. Drachenblut.

Sanguis Draconis.

Dæmonorops Draco *Blume.*

A brownish-red, opaque, brittle, inodorous, and insipid resin, affording a powder of a cinnabar color. Completely soluble in alcohol, but only partially soluble in ether, and the fixed and essential oils. It occurs in sticks of scarcely the thickness of a finger, covered with palm leaves, or comes in the form of cakes.

Resina Guajaci.

[GUAIAC]. Guajakharz.

[*Guaiacum Resin*].

Guajacum officinale *Linn.*

Guaiac occurs in globular pieces, from the size of a hazelnut to that of a walnut, or in irregular masses; covered on the outside with a greenish powder. It is friable, and has a yellowish-green, or nearly a chestnut-brown, and glassy fracture. It has a peculiar but rather feeble odor. It is colored green or blue by oxidizing agents. Soluble in alcohol, and in solution of caustic potassa.

Resina Jalapæ.

[RESIN OF JALAP]. Jalapenharz.

Take of Jalap Root, coarsely powdered, *one part*. . . 1
Pour upon it
Alcohol *four parts*, ... 4

and digest for twenty-four hours. Express when cold, and pour upon the residue *two parts* of Alcohol, and operate as before. Distill off the alcohol from the mixed and filtered tinctures by means of a steam-bath, and wash the resin with common hot water until the water runs off nearly colorless. Then heat the resin, by means of a steam-bath, until a small sample is found to be brittle, and readily pulverizable when cold. Afterwards form the resin into small rolls.

It has a shining fracture, is friable, and of a yellowish-brown color; completely soluble in alcohol. Ether dissolves only a small part of it.

It should be *cautiously* preserved.

Resini Pini.

[BURGUNDY PITCH]. Fichtenharz.

Resina Pini Burgundica. Pix alba.

From various species of Abies.

A yellow or yellowish-brown, opaque or translucent resin, having a shining fracture. It softens by the heat of the hand; has a terebinthinate odor, and is nearly wholly soluble in alcohol.

Resina Scammoniæ.

[RESIN OF SCAMMONY]. Scammoniaharz.

It is prepared from Scammony Root, like Resin of Jalap.

It has a greenish-brown color, a shining fracture, and dissolves completely in alcohol.

It should be *cautiously* preserved.

Rhizoma Calami.

[CALAMUS]. Kalmuswurzel.

[Sweet Flag]. Radix Calami.

Acorus Calamus *Linn.*

A subcylindrical, flattened rhizome, about two and half centimetres in breadth. Externally of a greenish, reddish, or brownish color; rather closely annulated, and marked with scars on the under surface, where the rootlets have been cut off. It is whitish internally, and has a spongy structure, owing to its very numerous air-passages. It has a strong, peculiar odor, and a bitter taste. The peeled rhizome only should be used for medicinal purposes.

It should be gathered in the latter part of autumn.

Rhizoma Caricis.

[SEA SEDGE]. Rothe Quecke.

Sandriedgraswurzel. Radix Caricis.

Carex arenaria *Linn.*

A very long, subcylindrical, somewhat flattened rhizome, about three millimetres thick; branched, and of a pale grayish-brown color, with remote nodes, at which only it is provided with lacerated, sheathing scales, and rootlets. The rhizome is filled with a white pith, and a dark-colored ring separates the bark (interrupted by the broad and circularly-arranged gaps), from the woody portion, which consists of dense woody bundles scattered through a scanty white cellular tissue. It causes a slight acridity in the fauces when chewed, and has a sweetish taste at first, afterwards somewhat bitter.

It should not be confounded with the rhizome of *Carex hirta* Linn., which is reddish-brown externally, and provided with rootlets between the nodes, and has a tough, white bark.

It should be gathered in the spring.

Rhizoma Chinæ.

[China Root]. Chinawurzel.

Radix Chinæ.

Smilax China ***Linn.***

The rhizomes are of various sizes and shapes, mostly oblong and curved, about twenty centimetres in length, and five centimetres in thickness; heavy and compact, freed from the rootlets, and partly from the outer bark. Externally of a reddish-brown, and internally of a reddish-white color, dotted with dark-colored specks, and provided with an abundance of starch. The root is mucilaginous when chewed, and has a somewhat harsh, but sweetish taste.

The light, spongy, as well as the paler rhizomes, should be rejected. Care should be taken that they are not contaminated with litharge, which is used to fill the perforations produced by worms.

Rhizoma Curcumæ.

[Turmeric]. Kurkuma.

Radix Curcumæ.

Curcuma longa ***Linn.,*** **et Curcuma viridiflora** ***Roxburgh.***

The rhizomes are either oval, of the size of a walnut (round Turmeric), or cylindrical, and about fourteen millimetres in thickness (long Turmeric). They are compact, heavy, somewhat horny; externally yellowish-brown, more or less annulated; on the transverse fracture flattish, orange-yellow, and provided with a darkish ring. They have a feeble ginger-like odor, and a burning, somewhat bitter taste when chewed, coloring the saliva yellow. A solution of the coloring matter has a bright-yellow color, which is changed to a brown by the alkalies, and also by boracic acid.

Rhizoma Filicis.

[MALE FERN]. Wurmfarnwurzel.

Radix Filicis maris.

Polystichum Filix mas *Roth.*

The rhizomes vary in length, and are about two and a half centimetres thick. They are fleshy when fresh; light, spongy, and internally of a green color, inclining to a cinnamon shade when dry; furnished with rather large, vascular bundles (fascicles), interruptedly arranged in a ring. The rhizomes are closely enveloped on their whole outer surface by the residue, or base of the footstalks (of the fronds), and numerous brown, chaff-like scales. The former arise obliquely, and point in one direction, are angular, fleshy, dark-brown externally, and green internally; these, together with the scales, characterize them from other similar-looking rhizomes. Their taste is sweetish-bitter, and their odor peculiar, and somewhat nauseous.

The rhizomes should be collected in the autumn, and not kept over a year.

The rhizomes, previous to the preparation of the powder, must be freed from the residual footstalks, scales, and rootlets, and, including the peeled footstalks, carefully dried, and the green powder preserved in well-closed vessels. Powder of a cinnamon-brown color must be rejected.

Rhizoma Galangæ.

[GALANGAL ROOT]. Galgant.

Radix Galangæ.

Alpinia officinarum *Fletcher Hance.*

The rhizome is as thick as a finger, about five centimetres long, cylindrical, short, somewhat branched, often geniculate; striated longitudinally; externally of a reddish-brown color, and marked with whitish, circular rings. Internally of a cinnamon color, and marked with a brown circle; it is very fibrous. It causes burning in the mouth when chewed, and has a somewhat bitter taste, and a peculiar odor.

Rhizoma Graminis.

[Couch-grass Root]. Queckenwurzel.

[*Quickens*]. ***Radix Graminis.***

Agropyrum repens ***Beauvois.***

A very long rhizome, about two millimetres in thickness, branched, hollow, cylindrical, and remotely jointed. It is furnished with radicels and scales only at the joints (nodes). It has a pale straw-color, and a sweet taste. Most of the cut roots occurring in commerce may be employed.

It should be gathered in the spring.

Rhizoma Imperatoriæ.

[Masterwort]. Meisterwurzel.

Radix Imperatoriæ.

Imperatoria Ostruthium *Linn.*

An elongated rhizome, nearly cylindrical, branched above, swollen and flattened, about two centimetres in breadth. Externally of a grayish-brown color, annulated, warty; internally fleshy, and of a pale lemon-yellow, with a thin woody portion. The bark and the broad pith are provided with large balsamiferous receptacles. It has a strong odor, and a bitter, burning taste.

The root may be gathered in the spring or autumn.

Rhizoma Iridis.

[Florentine Orris]. Veilchenwurzel.

[***Orris Root***]. ***Radix Iridis Florentinæ.***

Iris Florentina *Linn.*

Decorticated, somewhat flattened, solid, hard, and jointed rhizomes, of various lengths, nearly four centimetres in breadth; marked with scars on the lower surface where the rootlets have been cut off; they are often mixed with club-shaped branches. Orris root has a whitish color, and an odor resembling that of the violet.

Rhizoma Tormentillæ.

[TORMENTIL]. Tormentillwurzel.

[*Tormentilla Root*]. *Radix Tormentillæ.*

Potentilla Tormentilla *Sibthorp.*

The rhizome is knobby; its form is irregular, straight or crooked, with numerous heads, about two and a half centimetres in thickness, and eight centimetres in length; solid and hard. Externally of a dark red-brown color, gibbous, and marked with scars where the filiform rootlets have been cut off. Its color internally is brownish-red. It has a thin bark; is provided with a ring of whitish woody bundles, and a large pith. Its taste is strongly astringent.

The root should be gathered in the spring.

Rhizoma Veratri.

[WHITE HELLEBORE ROOT]. Weisse Nieswurzel.

Radix Veratri albi. Radix Hellebori albi.

Veratrum album *Linn.*

The rhizome is conical, about eight centimetres in length; at the upper part four to five centimetres in breadth, often many-headed. At the top it is tufted, caused by the cut edges of the leaves. It is externally of a blackish- or brownish-gray color, obscurely annulated, and marked with whitish scars where the numerous rootlets have been cut off. It has a dirty-white color internally, is hard, and exhibits a brown ring under the bark. It has a burning taste, and when rubbed excites very violent sneezing.

It should be *cautiously* preserved.

Rhizoma Zedoariæ.

[ZEDOARY ROOT]. Zittwerwurzel.

Radix Zedoariæ.

Curcuma-Zedoaria *Roscoe.*

The root (corm) is oval, annulated, about two and a half centimetres thick. The rootlets and outer bark are cut away, and it is divided transversely, and sometimes longitudinally. It is compact, tough, of a pale grayish-brown color, and provided with small, resiniferous glands. It causes burning in the mouth when chewed, has a bitterish taste, and a strong camphorous odor.

A light, worm-eaten article is to be rejected.

Rhizoma Zingiberis.

[GINGER]. Ingwer.

Radix Zingiberis.

Zingiber officinale *Roscoe.*

The rhizome is compact, heavy, two-ranked, and shortly branched, flattened, and about two centimetres broad. Either the entire surface is scraped, or only the two flat surfaces, and not the edges. Internally of a pale yellowish or whitish color, with a darker ring under the bark, and provided with small, very numerous, resiniferous receptacles. It has a somewhat fibrous fracture, and causes burning in the mouth when chewed. It has a peculiar, aromatic odor.

Very white ginger, bleached with lime, sometimes occurring in commerce, must not be employed.

Rotulæ Menthæ piperitæ.

[TROCHES OF PEPPERMINT]. Pfefferminzkuchen.

[***Peppermint Lozenges***].

Take of Sugar Lozenges *two hundred parts,*	200
Oil of Peppermint *one part,*	1
Alcohol *two parts.*	2

Pour the oil of peppermint and alcohol into a glass vessel, and turn it around so that the inner surface becomes moistened with the mixture. Then introduce the sugar lozenges, and shake them well around in the vessel to moisten them completely.

They should be preserved in well-closed vessels.

Saccharum.

[SUGAR]. Zucker.

Sugar should be very white and dry.

Saccharum Lactis.

[SUGAR OF MILK]. Milchzucker.

In cylindrical masses, or in the form of crusts, which consist of whitish, translucent, prismatic crystals, without odor. They have a sweetish taste, and are gritty between the teeth; soluble in six parts of cold water, but insoluble in alcohol.

Sandaraca.

[SANDARACH]. Sandarak.

Resina Sandaraca.

Callitris quadrivalis ***Ventenat.***

In longish, pale lemon-yellow, transparent grains (tears), dusted with a whitish powder, breaking with a glassy surface, and not becoming soft when chewed; of a bitterish taste. When heated, sandarach diffuses an agreeable odor, melts and inflames. It dissolves partly in cold alcohol, completely so in hot alcohol, and in oil of turpentine.

Santoninum.

[SANTONIN]. Santonin.

Acidum santonicum.

In small, shining, inodorous, crystalline scales; scarcely soluble in cold water, soluble in two hundred and fifty parts of boiling water, forty-four parts of cold, and in three parts of boiling alcohol, in seventy-five parts of cold, and two parts of hot ether, also in three parts of chloroform, forming neutral solutions. Santonin is nearly soluble in diluted acids, but freely so in solution of caustic potassa or soda, or lime-water. It is precipitated from the alkaline solutions by any of the acids. When cautiously heated, it melts at a temperature of 170° C., and, if allowed to cool slowly, forms a crystalline mass, but if it cools rapidly, the mass will be amorphous. When heated somewhat above the melting-point, it is sublimed partly without decomposition. It forms, with an alcoholic solution of caustic potassa, a scarlet liquid, which gradually becomes colorless. It assumes a yellow color on exposure to light.

It must be *cautiously* preserved and protected from the light.

Sapo domesticus.

[COMMON HARD SOAP]. Hausseife.

It should be as white and hard as possible, and dissolve in eight parts of boiling alcohol, which solution should form, on cooling, a nearly translucent, gelatinous mass.

Sapo jalapinus.

[JALAP SOAP]. Jalapenseife.

Take of Resin of Jalap, ... 4
Medicinal Soap, each, *four parts*, ... 4
dissolve them in
Diluted Alcohol *eight parts*, ... 8
and evaporate by means of a steam-bath, stirring constantly, to the consistence of a pilular mass, or so that the whole shall be *nine parts* by weight.

Jalap Soap has a brownish-gray color, and is soluble in alcohol.

Sapo medicatus.

[MEDICINAL SOAP]. Medicinische Seife.

Take of Solution of Caustic Soda *sixty parts*. . . 60

Pour it into a porcelain vessel, heat it by means of a steam-bath, and stir constantly, while adding gradually of

Provence Olive Oil *one hundred parts*. . . 100

Digest, stirring frequently, until a hard soap is formed.

Dissolve this soap in

Distilled Water *three hundred parts*, . . . 300

and add a solution of

Chloride of Sodium *twenty-five parts*, . . 25
Distilled Water *seventy-five parts*. . . . 75

Boil and stir until the soap has completely separated from the liquid portion, and, when it has cooled, wash it with Distilled Water. Dissolve it again in

Hot Distilled Water *sixty parts*, . . . 60

or sufficient to form a homogeneous mass, which pour, while still warm, into a box lined with a wet linen cloth. Remove the soap when cold, cut it into pieces, dry it in a moderately warm place, and lastly, convert into powder.

It should form a white powder, without a rancid odor, and be completely soluble in water, and in alcohol. The watery solution should not be altered by hydrosulphuric acid.

Sapo oleaceus.

[CASTILE SOAP]. Oelseife.

Sapo Hispanicus. Sapo Venetus.

Castile Soap should be white, hard, not becoming moist and tough when exposed to the air, and be free from rancidity. Completely soluble in alcohol, and in water.

Sapo terebinthinatus.

[TEREBINTHINATED SOAP]. Terpenthinölseife.

Balsamum vitæ externum.

Take of Castile Soap, powdered, ... 6
Oil of Turpentine, each, *six parts*, ... 6
Purified Carbonate of Potassium, in very fine powder, *one part*. 1

Mix them thoroughly, so as to form a mass of the consistence of an ointment.

It is white at first, changing to a yellowish color.

Sapo viridis.

[SOFT-SOAP]. Grüne Seife.

Sapo kalinus. Sapo niger.

A lubricous, soft, yellowish-green mass, of a nauseous smell.

Saturationes.

[NEUTRAL MIXTURES]. Saturationen.

When a Neutral Mixture (*Saturation*) is prescribed, without directions for its preparation, *Solution of Citrate of Sodium* (*Potio Riveri*), is always dispensed.

When a Neutral Mixture is prescribed, for which the acid and the alkaline base are especially given, it should be prepared like Solution of Citrate of Sodium (*Potio Riveri*).

Sebum.

[SUET OR TALLOW]. Talg.

Bos Taurus *Linn.* **Ovis Aries** *Linn.*

A solid, white, fatty substance, of a peculiar smell, melting at a temperature of between 45° and 50° C.

Rancid Suet should be rejected.

Secale cornutum.

[Ergot]. Mutterkorn.

Claviceps purpurea *Tulasne.*

The grains of Ergot consist of the sterile beds (*Stromata sterilia*) of fungus spores. They are obtusely-triangular, generally curved, tapering towards both ends, or sometimes only towards the upper extremity, and are marked with three furrows. They have a violet-blackish color, often covered by a bloom, paler internally, and not unfrequently provided at the apex with a soft, dull-white appendage (*calyptra*). The grains are about two and a half centimetres long, and three millimetres broad. Their odor is nauseous.

Ergot should be collected only from the spikelets of rye (*Secale cereale* Linn.), and in its dry state, preserved in well-closed vessels, and, when possible, be renewed every year. Worm-eaten, mouldy, rancid—and ergot which has an ammoniacal odor—should be rejected.

Semen Colchici.

[Colchicum Seeds]. Zeitlosensamen.

Colchicum autumnale *Linn.*

The fully ripe seeds of colchicum are subglobose, upwards of two millimetres thick, and horny; externally dark-brown, pitted, and, if not too old, somewhat glutinous; internally of a pale-gray color. They have a very bitter, nauseous taste.

The seeds should be gathered in the beginning of summer, *cautiously* preserved, but not kept longer than a year.

Semen Cydoniæ.

[Quince Seeds]. Quittensamen.

Quittenkörner.

Cydonia vulgaris *Persoon.*

Quince seeds are wedge-shaped, angular, or compressed, about six millimetres in length, of a chestnut-brown color, and covered with a whitish, opaque coat, abounding in mucilage; a number generally adhering together. They swell up in water, and owing to their softened, mucilaginous coat, become lubricous. They should be free from the well-known apple, pear, and grape seeds.

Semen Fœni Græci.

[FENUGREEK SEEDS]. Bockshornsamen.

Trigonella Fœnum Græcum *Linn.*

Fenugreek seeds are very hard, nearly rhomboidal-four-cornered, obliquely truncated at both ends, yellowish-brown, and about three millimetres in length, with hook-shaped embryo, and a strongly elevated radicle under the shell (testa). They have a disagreeable, strongly melilot-like odor, and a mucilaginous, bitter taste when chewed.

Semen Hyoscyami.

[HYOSCYAMUS SEEDS]. Bilsensamen.

Hyoscyamus niger *Linn.*

Hyoscyamus seeds are very small, compressed, nearly kidney-shaped, finely pitted, and grayish-brown; internally whitish, and have an oily, bitter taste.

The seeds should be perfectly ripe.

They are to be *cautiously* preserved, but not kept longer than a year.

Semen Lini.

[FLAXSEED. LINSEED]. Leinsamen.

Linum usitatissimum *Linn.*

The seeds are ovate, compressed, about four millimetres long, of a chestnut-brown color, shining; when softened by water, become lubricous. They have an oily, mucilaginous taste. They should not be preserved longer than a year, and be free from the seeds of *Lolium arvensis* Schrader.

The seeds of the plant cultivated in Germany should be used in the preparation of flaxseed meal.

Semen Myristicæ.

[NUTMEG]. Muskatnuss.

Nux moschata.

Myristica fragrans *Houttuyn.*

The kernel is oval, about two and a half centimetres long, reticulated externally, frequently dusted with a white powder. Internally it is pale-brown. The dark, orange-yellow projecting ridges of the inner integument give it a marbled appearance. It has an aromatic odor and taste.

Mouldy and worm-eaten nutmegs, as well as the oblong and longer kernels of *Myristica fatua* Houtt., which have a weaker odor and taste, should be rejected.

Semen Papaveris.

[POPPY SEEDS]. Mohnsamen.

[***Maw Seeds***].

Papaver somniferum *Linn.*

Poppy seeds are kidney-shaped, reticulated-pitted, whitish, and have a sweetish, oily taste.

Old and rancid seeds should be rejected.

Semen Quercus tostum.

[ROASTED ACORNS]. Eichelkaffee.

[***Acorn Coffee***].

Acorns are roasted in a closed, hollow, iron cylinder over a fire, the cylinder being turned round, until they have acquired a brown color, and are then, upon cooling, reduced to a coarse powder.

They form a brownish powder of a somewhat pyroligneous odor, resembling roasted coffee, and of scarcely an astringent taste.

Semen Sinapis.

[Black Mustard Seed]. Schwarzer Senfsamen.

Brassica nigra *Koch.*

Black Mustard Seeds are roundish, one millimetre in thickness, finely pitted, externally of a rust-brown color, internally yellow. They afford a yellowish-green powder, which, when moistened with water, exhales a strong, pungent odor, and when chewed has at first a bitter, oily taste, afterwards causes a sharp burning in the mouth.

The seeds should not be adulterated with the seeds of *Brassica Rapa* Linn., which are one and a half times larger, also smoother, of a dark-brown color, and less pungent; nor with the larger seeds of the black variety of *Sinapis alba* Linn.

Powdered Mustard should always be kept ready, freshly prepared.

Semen Stramonii.

[Stramonium Seeds]. Stechapfelsamen.

Semen Daturæ.

Datura Stramonium *Linn.*

Stramonium Seeds are kidney-shaped, compressed, lightly pitted; externally dull black, and internally white; about two millimetres long, and but a little more in width. They have a disagreeable, bitter taste.

The seeds should be fully ripe, and be *cautiously* preserved.

Semen Strychni.

[Nux Vomica]. Krähenaugen.

Brechnuss. Strychnossamen. Nux vomica.

Strychnos Nux vomica *Linn.*

The seeds are disk-shaped, circular, about two and a half centimetres in diameter, umbilicated in the centre, clothed with a coat of very dense, silky, appressed hairs of a yellowish-gray color. The seeds are horny, split and whitish within; of a very bitter taste.

The commercial powder should not be employed.

Nux Vomica must be *cautiously* preserved.

Serum Lactis.

[WHEY]. Molken.

Serum Lactis dulce.

Take of Fresh Cow's Milk *two hundred parts*, . . 200
Essence of Rennet *one part*. 1

Mix thoroughly, heat them to a temperature ranging between 35° and 40° C., set aside, and after complete coagulation of the milk, separate, by straining, the whey from the curd (casein).

Whey should have a yellowish-white color, and be free from acidity.

Serum Lactis acidum.

[ACID WHEY. SOUR WHEY]. Saure Molken.

Take of Fresh Cow's Milk *one hundred parts*. . . 100
Heat it to the boiling point, and add of
Bitartrate of Potassium *one part*. . . . 1

After complete coagulation, strain the cold whey from the curd, and filter.

It has an acidulous taste, and is somewhat turbid.

Serum Lactis aluminatum.

[ALUM WHEY]. Alaunmolken.

Alum Whey is prepared like Acid Whey, except in place of Bitartrate of Potassium, there is employed
Alum, powdered, *one part*. 1

Serum Lactis tamarindinatum.

[TAMARIND WHEY]. Tamarindenmolken.

Tamarind Whey is prepared like Acid Whey, except in place of Bitartrate of Potassium, there is employed
Crude Tamarind Pulp *four parts*. . . . 4

It has a reddish-brown color.

Sinapismus.

[MUSTARD POULTICE]. Senfteig.

Take of Black Mustard Seeds, powdered, *a desired quantity.*
Mix it with an *equal quantity* of
Common Water,
and form a poultice of a somewhat soft consistence.

It is prepared only when wanted for dispensing.

Species aromaticæ.

[AROMATIC SPECIES OR HERBS]. Aromatische Kräuter.

Take of Peppermint,	2
Rosemary Leaves,	2
Wild Thyme,	2
Sweet Marjoram,	2
Lavender Flowers, each, *two parts,*	2
Cloves,	1
Cubebs, each, *one part.*	1

Having them, separately, finely cut and bruised, remove the fine dust and mix.

It should be preserved in a closed vessel.

Species ad Decoctum Lignorum.

[WOOD TEA]. Holzthee.

Take of Guaiacum Wood, rasped, *four parts,*	4
Burdock Root, cut,	2
Rest-harrow Root, cut, each, *two parts,*	2
Peeled Liquorice Root, cut,	1
Sassafras Wood, cut, each, *one part.*	1

Mix them.

Species emollientes.

[EMOLLIENT SPECIES OR HERBS]. Erweichende Kräuter.

Take of Marshmallow Leaves,	1
Common Mallow Leaves,	1
Melilot,	1
German Chamomile,	1
Flaxseed, each, *one part.*	1

Bruise them to a coarse powder, and mix.

Species ad Gargarisma.

[TEA FOR GARGLING]. Species zum Gurgeln.

Take of Marshmallow Leaves,
Elder Flowers,
Common Mallow Flowers, each, *equal parts.*
Cut and mix them.

Species laxantes St. Germain.

[ST. GERMAIN TEA]. Saint-Germainthee.

Take of	Senna, exhausted by alcohol, *sixteen parts,*	16
	Elder Flowers *ten parts,*	10
	Fennel Seeds,	5
	Anise, each, *five parts.*	5

Cut, bruise, and mix them.
When it is dispensed, add of

	Bitartrate of Potassium *three parts.*	3

Species pectorales.

[PECTORAL TEA]. Brustthee.

Species ad Infusum pectorale.

Take of	Marshmallow Root, cut, *eight parts,*	8
	Peeled Liquorice Root, cut, *three parts,*	3
	Florentine Orris, cut, *one part,*	1
	Coltsfoot, cut, *four parts,*	4
	Common Mullein Flowers, cut,	2
	Star-anise, bruised, each, *two parts.*	2

Mix them.

Species pectorales cum Fructibus.

[PECTORAL TEA WITH FRUITS]. Brustthee mit Früchten.

Take of	Pectoral Tea *sixteen parts,*	16
	St. John's Bread, cut, *six parts,*	6
	Pearl Barley *four parts,*	4
	Figs, cut, *three parts.*	3

Mix them.

Spiritus.

[ALCOHOL]. Weingeist.

Spiritis Vini rectificatissimus. Alcohol Vini.

A clear, colorless liquid, entirely free from fusel oil, wholly volatile, and neutral in its reaction. Its specific gravity varies from 0.830 to 0.834, which correspond to from 91 to 90 per cent. of absolute alcohol by volume.

Spiritus æthereus.

[SPIRIT OF ETHER]. Hoffmannstropfen.

[***Hoffman's Anodyne***]. ***Aetherweingeist. Liquor anodynus mineralis Hoffmanni.***

Take of Ether *one part*, ... 1
Alcohol *three parts*. 3

Mix them.

A clear, colorless liquid, with a specific gravity of from 0.808 to 0.812.

It should be preserved in well-closed vessels.

Spiritus Ætheris chlorati.

[SPIRIT OF CHLORIC ETHER]. Versüsster Salzgeist.

Spiritus Salis dulcis. Spiritus muriatico-æthereus.

Take of Black Oxide of Manganese, broken into pieces of the size of a hazelnut, *a sufficient quantity*.

Fill with these pieces a flask (or matrass) up to the neck. The flask must have a capacity of *one hundred and twenty parts* of water, by weight. Pour upon the manganese, but without covering the whole of it,

Crude Hydrochloric Acid *six parts*, ... 6
Alcohol *twenty-four parts*, ... 24

previously mixed; and, having connected the flask with a refrigeratory, distill *twenty-five parts*. Then neutralize the distillate by means of slaked lime, and redistill, with a gentle heat, *twenty-one parts*.

It forms a clear and colorless liquid, free from acid, with a specific gravity of from 0.838 to 0.842.

Spiritus Ætheris nitrosi.

[SPIRIT OF NITROUS ETHER]. Versüsster Salpetergeist.

[*Sweet Spirit of Nitre*]. *Spiritus nitroso-œthereus. Spiritus nitrico-œthereus. Spiritus Nitri dulcis.*

Take of Alcohol *forty-eight parts*, ... 48
Pure Nitric Acid *twelve parts*. 12
Introduce them into a glass retort, and distill off *forty parts*. 40

Add to the distillate, while stirring, a sufficient quantity of Magnesia to neutralize the acid. Set it aside for twenty-four hours, then pour off the clear liquid, and redistill it by means of a steam-bath.

Spirit of Nitrous Ether is clear, of an agreeable etheral odor, nearly colorless, as free as possible from acid, and has a specific gravity of between 0.840 and 0.850.

It should be preserved in small, completely-filled, well-closed bottles, and kept in a cool place.

Spiritus Angelicæ compositus.

[COMPOUND SPIRIT OF ANGELICA]. Zusammengesetzter Engelwurzelspiritus.

In place of Spiritus theriacalis.

Take of Garden Angelica Root, cut, *sixteen parts*, . . 16
Valerian Root, cut, ... 4
Juniper Berries, bruised, each, *four parts*. . 4
Introduce them into a retort; pour upon them
Alcohol *seventy-five parts*, ... 75
Common Water *one hundred and twenty-five parts*, 125
and macerate for twenty-four hours.
Then distill off *one hundred parts*, ... 100
in which dissolve
Camphor *two parts*, ... 2
and lastly, filter.

A clear, colorless liquid.

Spiritus camphoratus.

[SPIRIT OF CAMPHOR]. Kampferspiritus.

Take of Camphor *one part*, ... 1
dissolve it in
Alcohol *seven parts*, ... 7
and add of
Distilled Water *two parts*. 2

Spirit of Camphor is clear and colorless.

Spiritus Cochleariæ.

[SPIRIT OF COMMON SCURVY-GRASS]. Löffelkrautspiritus.

Take of the fresh flowering Common Scurvy-Grass *eight parts*. 8
Pour upon it
Alcohol, ... 3
Common Water, each, *three parts*, . . . 3
and distill off *four parts*. 4

A clear, colorless liquid.

Spiritus dilutus.

[DILUTED ALCOHOL]. Verdünnter Spiritus.

Verdünnter Weingeist. Spiritus Vini rectificatus.

Take of Alcohol *seven parts*, ... 7
Distilled Water *three parts*. 3

Mix them.

Diluted Alcohol is clear and colorless. It has a specific gravity of from 0.892 to 0.893, and contains from sixty-nine to sixty-eight per cent. of absolute alcohol by volume.

Spiritus Formicarum.

[SPIRIT OF ANTS]. Ameisenspiritus.

Take of Ants, recently gathered and bruised, *ten parts,*	10
Alcohol, ...	15
Common Water, each, *fifteen parts.* . . .	15
Macerate for two days, then distill off *twenty parts.* .	20

A clear, colorless liquid, which reddens blue test-paper. Twenty parts, mixed with one part of solution of subacetate of lead, should form a mixture almost entirely filled with feathery crystals.

Spiritus Juniperi.

[SPIRIT OF JUNIPER]. Wachholderspiritus.

Take of Juniper Berries, bruised, *five parts,* . . .	5
Alcohol, ...	15
Common Water, each, *fifteen parts.* . . .	15
Macerate for twenty-four hours, then distill off *twenty parts.*	20

Spirit of Juniper is clear and colorless.

Spiritus Lavandulæ.

[SPIRIT OF LAVENDER]. Lavendelspiritus.

It is prepared from Lavender Flowers, like Spirit of Juniper.

Spirit of Lavender is clear and colorless.

Spiritus Melissæ compositus.

[COMPOUND SPIRIT OF BALM]. Karmelitergeist.

Take of Balm Leaves *fourteen parts*, ... 14
Lemon Peel *twelve parts*, ... 12
Coriander Seeds, ... 6
Nutmeg, each, *six parts*, ... 6
Cassia Bark, ... 3
Cloves, each, *three parts*. 3

Having cut and bruised the ingredients, pour upon them

Alcohol *one hundred and fifty parts*, ... 150
Common Water *two hundred and fifty parts*, . 250

and distill off *two hundred parts*. 200

Compound Spirit of Balm is clear and colorless.

Spiritus Menthæ crispæ Anglicus.

[ENGLISH ESSENCE OF CURLED-MINT]. Englische Krauseminzessenz.

Take of Oil of Curled-mint *one part*, ... 1
Alcohol *nine parts*. 9

Mix them.

It is clear and colorless.

Spiritus Menthæ piperitæ Anglicus.

[ENGLISH ESSENCE OF PEPPERMINT]. Englische Pfefferminzessenz.

Take of Oil of Peppermint *one part*, ... 1
Alcohol *nine parts*. 9

Mix them.

It is clear and colorless.

Spiritus Rosmarini.

[SPIRIT OF ROSEMARY]. Rosmarinspiritus.

Spiritus Anthos.

It is prepared from Rosemary Leaves, like Spirit of Juniper. Spirit of Rosemary is clear and colorless.

Spiritis Saponatus.

[SPIRIT OF SOAP]. Seifenspiritus.

Take of Castile Soap, in shavings, *one part*. 1
Dissolve by digestion, with a gentle heat, in
Alcohol *three parts*, ... 3
Rose Water *two parts*, ... 2
and filter.

Spirit of Soap is clear, with a yellowish color.
It should be preserved in not too cold a place.

Spiritus Serpylli.

[SPIRIT OF WILD THYME]. Quendelspiritus.

It is prepared from Wild Thyme, like Spirit of Juniper.
It is clear and colorless.

Spiritus Sinapis.

[SPIRIT OF MUSTARD]. Senfspiritus.

Take of Oil of Mustard *one part*, ... 1
Alcohol *fifty parts*. 50
Mix them.
It should be *cautiously* preserved in well-closed vessels.

Spongiæ ceratæ.

[WAXED SPONGE. SPONGE TENT]. Wachsschwämme.

It is prepared by freeing finely-porous sponge from foreign matter, drying and cutting it in proper shape, dipping the pieces in melted yellow wax, forcibly compressing them between heated plates, and, when cold, freeing them from superfluous wax.

Spongiæ compressæ.

[COMPRESSED SPONGE]. Presschwamm.

It is prepared by carefully freeing finely-porous, select sponge from shells and gravel, cutting it into longish pieces, which are moistened with hot water, and each wound closely with pack-thread, to compress them into cylinders about as long as a finger. These are dried and preserved with their binding threads.

Stibium sulfuratum aurantiacum.

[GOLDEN SULPHURET OF ANTIMONY]. Goldschwefel.

Sulphur Stibiatum aurantiacum. Sulphur auratum Antimonii.

A very fine, orange-yellow, inodorous powder, insoluble in water, and alcohol, but soluble in hot concentrated hydrochloric acid, leaving a residue of sulphur. On heating in a glass tube, it yields sublimed sulphur, and a residue of black tersulphuret of antimony.

It is completely soluble in solution of caustic potassa. It should dissolve in from sixty to eighty parts of water of ammonia, leaving but a small amount of a residue, which is soluble in tartaric acid. When triturated with distilled water, the filtered liquid should have no acid taste, and should not be rendered turbid by nitrate of silver. Triturated with an equal part of bicarbonate of sodium and some water, the filtered liquid does not assume a yellow turbidity on the addition of hydrochloric acid in excess.

It should be protected from the light, and preserved in well-closed vessels.

Stibium sulfuratum crudum.

[Black Sulphuret of Antimony]. Schwefelspiessglanz.

[*Crude Antimony*]. *Antimonium crudum.*

In heavy, blackish-gray, shining lumps, soiling the fingers, and having a radiated, crystalline fracture. When heated with hydrochloric acid, it is decomposed with the evolution of hydrosulphuric acid gas.

It should be as free as possible from arsenic, lead, and copper.

Powdered, it should almost entirely dissolve when boiled with ten parts of hydrochloric acid. One part of this clear, decanted solution, when mixed with an equal volume of alcohol, should form but a slightly turbid mixture, which, when treated with an excess of water of ammonia, should not yield a very blue filtrate. Another part of the same solution, mixed with hydrochloric acid, and a small quantity of protochloride of tin added, must not assume a deep-brown color on being heated.

Stibium sulfuratum lævigatum.

[Levigated Black Sulphuret of Antimony]. Fein zerriebenes Schwefelspiessglanz.

Stibium sulphuratum nigrum lævigatum.

It should be entirely free from arsenic, and as much as possible so from lead and copper.

Stibium sulfuratum rubeum.

[Kermes Mineral]. Mineralkermes.

[*Oxysulphuret of Antimony*]. *Sulphur stibiatum rubeum. Kermes minerale.*

Take of Commercial Carbonate of Sodium *twenty-five parts*. 25

Dissolve it in

Common Water *two hundred and fifty parts*, . 250

previously heated to the boiling point in an iron kettle, and, while stirring, add of

Levigated Black Sulphuret of Antimony *one part*. 1

Boil for two hours, and constantly replace the water that is evaporated; then filter the boiling hot solution into a vessel containing a little Hot Water. After cooling, collect the precipitate on a filter, and wash it on the same with Distilled Water until the liquid runs off colored, and no longer affects red test-paper. Finally, express between folds of bibulous paper, and dry it in a dark, luke-warm place (25° C.), rub it to fine powder, and preserve it in well-closed vessels, which are to be protected from the light.

Kermes Mineral is a very fine, reddish-brown powder, containing minute crystals, which may be detected by means of a lens.

Stipites Dulcamaræ.

[BITTERSWEET]. Bittersüssstengel.

Solanum Dulcamara ***Linn.***

The stems or twigs of Bittersweet are straggling and often twining, from four to eight millimetres in thickness, nearly five-angled, marked with scattered scars left by the fallen leaves. They are more or less warty, striated or furrowed longitudinally, and most generally hollow. The periderm is greenish or brownish-yellow, and separates readily from the thin bark, which is at first of a green, and finally of a whitish color. The woody portion is very porous, and at first green, changing to a yellowish color, and frequently furnished with concentric rings. The bark has a bitter, and the wood a sweet taste.

The twigs of the two or three years old plants should be gathered in autumn, when they have shed their leaves. They should not be confounded with the stems of *Lonicera Periclymenum* L., which are cylindrical, and marked with opposite scars of the fallen leaves.

Strychninum.

[STRYCHNIA]. Strychnin.

In small, hard, columnar crystals, of a very bitter taste; scarcely soluble in cold, and but slightly in boiling water; almost insoluble in ether, and in absolute alcohol; it dissolves a little more readily in diluted alcohol. One hundred parts of alcohol, of the specific gravity 0.889, dissolve five parts of strychnia, forming a solution of an alkaline reaction, and which, even though largely diluted, possesses a bitter, afterwards disagreeable, taste.

Strychnia, dissolved in concentrated sulphuric acid without the aid of heat, yields, on the addition of a small crystal of bichromate of potassium, a blue or violet color, speedily passing through red to green. The above alcoholic solution of Strychnia affords, on the addition of solution of caustic potassa, a precipitate which is insoluble in an excess of the alkaline solution. Salts of Strychnia, on which has been poured concentrated nitric acid, must only become yellow when heated. Strychnia should form, with dilute nitric acid, a colorless, and in no case a red, solution.

It should be *very cautiously* preserved.

Strychninum nitricum.

[NITRATE OF STRYCHNIA]. Salpetersaures Strychnin.

In small, hard crystals, frequently of a silky lustre; soluble in sixty parts of cold, and in three parts of boiling water; very sparingly soluble in absolute alcohol, more readily in diluted alcohol. The solutions are neutral, and have a very bitter taste.

It behaves in the presence of reagents like Strychnia.

It should be *very cautiously* preserved.

Styrax liquidus.

[LIQUID STORAX]. Flüssiger Storax.

Liquidambar orientale ***Miller.***

An opaque mass, of a more or less gray color, and the consistence of rather thick [European] turpentine. It contains sometimes a little water, and has a peculiar pleasant odor. It is almost entirely soluble in alcohol.

Succinum.

[AMBER]. Bernstein.

In yellow, or yellowish-brown, transparent or opaque pieces. They are brittle, have a conchoidal, shining fracture, and are scarcely soluble in alcohol, ether, the fixed and essential oils.

Succus Juniperi inspissatus.

[EXTRACT OF JUNIPER BERRIES]. Wachholdermus.

Roob Juniperi.

Pour upon *one part* of fresh Juniper berries, bruised, *four parts* of Hot Common Water, and when cold, express moderately. Allow the liquid to settle, then strain and evaporate it to the consistence of a *thin* extract.

It is brown, and forms a turbid solution with water.

Succus Liquiritiæ crudus.

[LIQUORICE]. Lakriz.

[***Crude Extract of Liquorice***]. ***Extractum Glycyrrhizæ crudum.***

Glycyrrhiza glabra *Linn.*

Liquorice occurs in the form of rolls, which are nearly cylindrical, about fifteen centimetres in length, and about two and a half centimetres in thickness, of a brownish-black, shining color; brittle when cold, and breaking with a black, glossy fracture. It has a sweet taste, with scarcely any acridity. It dissolves largely in water.

Succus Liquiritiæ depuratus.

[REFINED LIQUORICE]. Gereinigter Lakrizensaft.

[***Purified Extract of Liquorice***]. ***Extractum Glycyrrhizæ depuratum.***

Liquorice (crude extract) is introduced into an upright cask, placed in layers, with washed straw between each layer, and covered with Cold Common Water, and allowed to macerate for thirty-six hours. The liquid is then drawn off through a faucet, and the maceration is repeated, as often as necessary, with fresh portions of Water. The strained and perfectly clear liquids are then evaporated, by means of a steam-bath, to the consistence of a *thick* extract.

Refined Liquorice has a brown color, and forms a clear solution with water.

Succus Sambuci inspissatus.

[EXTRACT OF ELDER BERRIES]. Fliedermus.

[*Inspissated Elder Berry Juice*].

Heat fresh, ripe Elder Berries, with constant stirring, until they burst open, then express. Allow the expressed juice to settle, then strain and evaporate it to the consistence of a *thick* extract. To *twelve parts*, . . . 12
of this inspissated juice, while still warm, add of
White Sugar, powdered, *one part*. . . . 1

Care should be taken that it be not contaminated with copper, which may be detected by means of a polished iron blade.

It has a reddish-brown color, and a sweetish, acidulous taste. It forms almost a clear solution with water.

Sulfur depuratum.

[WASHED SULPHUR]. Gereinigte Schwefelblumen.

[*Washed or Purified Flowers of Sulphur*]. *Flores Sulphuris loti.*

Take of Sublimed Sulphur, passed through a sieve, *twelve parts*, ... 12
Distilled Water *eight parts*, ... 8
Water of Ammonia *one part*. 1

Mix so that they form a pasty mass, which digest for three days, stirring occasionally; then introduce it into a conical linen strainer, and wash thoroughly with distilled water. Lastly dry, and pass it through a sieve.

Washed Sulphur is a fine, dry, inodorous, and tasteless powder, of a lemon-yellow color. When heated it volatilizes, leaving but a very small residue. Entirely soluble in solution of caustic potassa. When moistened with water, it must not redden blue test-paper. Digested with water of ammonia, it yields a filtrate which must not be affected by hydrochloric acid in excess.

It should be preserved in a well-closed vessel.

Sulfur iodatum.

[IODIDE OF SULPHUR]. Jodschwefel.

Take of Washed Sulphur *one part*, ... 1
Iodine *four parts*. 4

Mix by rubbing them together; introduce the mixture into a flask, and apply a gentle heat until it melts into a uniform mass, which, when cold, reduce to powder.

Iodide of Sulphur has a blackish-gray color, metallic lustre, and volatilizes entirely by heat.

It should be *cautiously* preserved in a well-closed vessel.

Sulfur præcipitatum.

[PRECIPITATED SULPHUR]. Schwefelmilch.

[*Milk of Sulphur*]. *Lac Sulphuris.*

A very fine, yellowish-white, nearly inodorous powder. It is not gritty between the fingers, and leaves but a small residue when volatilized by heat.

It must not redden moistened blue test-paper. Water, hydrochloric acid, or water of ammonia, digested with it, and filtered, should not on evaporation leave any residue.

It should be preserved in a well-closed vessel.

Sulfur sublimatum.

[SUBLIMED SULPHUR]. Schwefelblumen.

[*Flowers of Sulphur*]. *Flores Sulphuris.*

Care should be taken that it be but slightly contaminated with selenium and arsenic. Water of ammonia digested with it, and filtered, should not be rendered turbid, or but very slightly so, on the addition of hydrochloric acid in excess.

Summitates Sabinæ.

[SAVINE]. Sadebaumspitzen.

[*Savine Tops*]. *Herba Sabinæ.*

Sabina officinalis *Garcke.*

The coarctate (contracted) branches, with very short, stiff leaves, which are furnished with a sunken gland on their dorsal side. The younger leaves, in four rows, are imbricated, rhombic, and somewhat obtuse; the older ones are more or less separated, spreading, and pointed. They have a strong, disagreeable, and persistent odor, and a nauseous, resinous, bitter taste. The branches should not be confounded with those of Red Cedar (*Sabina Virginiana*, Berg.), which are more spreading, and diffuse a feebler odor.

They should be *cautiously* preserved, but not kept longer than a year.

The tops of the shrub, cultivated in Germany, of the plant indigenous in Southern Europe, may be gathered in April and May, and employed.

Syrupi.

[SYRUPS]. Syrupe.

Syrups are prepared, when not otherwise ordered, by dissolving White Sugar in the clear liquid, with the aid of heat, and raising the temperature to the boiling-point.

The strained syrups, when entirely cold, are introduced into perfectly dry vessels, well closed, and kept in a cold place.

They should be all clear, with the exception of Syrup of Almonds, have no deposit, and be free from fermentation.

Syrupus Althææ.

[SYRUP OF MARSHMALLOW]. Eibischsaft.

Take of Marshmallow Root, cut, *one part*. 1

Wash it with cold distilled water; then pour upon it

Cold Distilled Water *twenty parts*, ... 20

macerate for two hours, and strain through a woolen cloth without pressure. In *fifteen parts* 15

of the strained liquid, dissolve

White Sugar *twenty-four parts*, ... 24

so that a syrup may be formed.

Syrup of Marshmallow is clear, with a slight yellow color.

Syrupus Amygdalarum.

[SYRUP OF ALMONDS]. Mandelsyrup.

Syrupus emulsivus.

Take of Sweet Almonds, decorticated (blanched), *four parts*, ... 4
Bitter Almonds, decorticated, *one part*. . . 1
Rub them to a very smooth paste with a little water, and gradually add of
Distilled Water *eleven parts*, ... 11
Orange-Flower Water *one part*, ... 1
express forcibly, strain through a woolen cloth, and dissolve, with a very gentle heat, in *eleven parts* . . 11
of the strained liquid,
White Sugar, powdered, *twenty parts*. . . 20
Syrup of Almonds is turbid and whitish.

Syrupus Aurantii Corticis.

[SYRUP OF ORANGE PEEL]. Pomeranzenschalensyrup.

Take of Orange Peel, cut, *two parts*, ... 2
Genuine White Wine *fourteen parts*, ... 14
digest for two days in a closed vessel, then express and filter.
Dissolve in *eleven parts* 11
of the filtered liquid
White Sugar *eighteen parts*, ... 18
so as to form a syrup.
Syrup of Orange Peel has a yellowish-brown color.

Syrupus Aurantii Florum.

[SYRUP OF ORANGE-FLOWERS]. Pomeranzenblüthensyrup.

In place of Syrupus Capillorum Veneris.

Take of White Sugar *nine parts*, ... 9
dissolve it in
Orange-Flower Water *five parts*, ... 5
so as to form a syrup.
The Syrup is colorless.

Syrupus Balsami Peruviani.

[SYRUP OF BALSAM OF PERU]. Perubalsamsyrup.

Syrupus balsamicus.

Take of Balsam of Peru *one part*, ... 1
Distilled Water *eleven parts*, ... 11
digest for several hours in a closed vessel, with frequent agitation. When cold, dissolve in *ten parts* . . . 10
of the decanted and filtered liquid,
White Sugar *eighteen parts*, ... 18
so as to form a syrup.

The Syrup has a yellowish color.

Syrupus Cerasi.

[SYRUP OF CHERRIES]. Kirschsyrup.

Take of fresh dark-purple Sour Cherries *a desired quantity*.

Bruise them, together with the seeds, and set aside for three days; then express the juice, and set it aside until it has become clear by fermentation.

Dissolve in *five parts* 5
of the filtered juice,
White Sugar *nine parts*, ... 9
so as to form a syrup.

The Syrup has dark purple color.

Syrupus Chamomillæ.

[SYRUP OF CHAMOMILE]. Kamillensyrup.

Take of German Chamomile *three parts*, ... 3
Boiling Distilled Water *fifteen parts*. . . . 15

Set aside for a few hours in a closed vessel, and dissolve in *ten parts* 10
of the filtered liquid,
White Sugar *eighteen parts*, ... 18
so as to form a syrup.

Syrup of Chamomile has a yellowish-brown color.

Syrupus Cinnamomi.

[Syrup of Cinnamon]. Zimmtsyrup.

Take of Cassia Bark, coarsely powdered, *two parts*, . 2
Spirituous Cinnamon Water *twelve parts*, . . 12
Rose Water *two parts*. 2
Digest for two days, in a closed vessel, and filter.
Dissolve in *eleven parts* 11
of the filtered liquid,
White Sugar *eighteen parts*, ... 18
so as to form a syrup.

Syrup of Cinnamon has a reddish-brown color.

Syrupus Croci.

[Syrup of Saffron]. Safransyrup.

Take of Saffron *one part*,. 1
Genuine White Wine *twenty-four parts*. . . 24
Macerate for thirty-six hours in a closed vessel, and dissolve in *twenty-two parts* 22
of the filtered liquid,
White Sugar *thirty-six parts*, ... 36
so as to form a syrup.

.It has a saffron-yellow color.

Syrupus Ferri iodati.

[Syrup of Iodide of Iron]. Eisenjodürsyrup.

Take of Powdered Iron *two parts*. 2
Introduce it into a sufficiently large flask, containing
Distilled Water *thirty parts*, ... 30
and add gradually of
Iodine *four parts*. 4

Dissolve by gently agitating the flask, and, if necessary, by the application of a gentle heat. Then filter the solution into a porcelain capsule, containing
White Sugar, powdered, *sixty parts*, ... 60
and add Distilled Water through the filter to wash it and the undissolved iron well. Dissolve the sugar with a very gentle heat, and evaporate the liquid, by means of a steam-bath, so that *one hundred parts* . . . 100
shall remain.

Freshly prepared Syrup of Iodide of Iron is nearly colorless, but it changes to a yellowish color. It contains five per cent. of iodide of iron.

It should be preserved in a small, very tightly-closed bottle, which should contain a piece of bright iron wire. The vessel should be kept in a light place.

Syrupus Ferri oxydati solubilis.

[Syrup of Oxide of Iron]. Eisensyrup.

Take the mass (*one hundred parts*) which is procured in the preparation of Saccharated Oxide of Iron by the mixing of the moist precipitate with sugar; and digest, by means of a steam-bath, for two hours, adding water which is lost by evaporation. When the mass has cooled, add of

Simple Syrup *a sufficient quantity* to make the whole amount to *three hundred parts*. . . 300

It forms a clear syrup of a dark red-brown color, and of a sweet, mildly ferruginous taste. When mixed with five parts of water it deposits no sediment. It contains one per cent. of iron.

Syrupus Fœniculi.

[Syrup of Fennel]. Fenchelsaft.

Take of Fennel Seeds, bruised, *two parts*, . . . 2
Boiling Distilled Water *twelve parts*, . . 12
and digest for three hours in a closed vessel.

Dissolve in *ten parts* 10
of the filtered liquid,
White Sugar *eighteen parts*, ... 18
so as to form a syrup.

Syrup of Fennel has a brownish-yellow color.

Syrupus gummosus.

[Syrup of Gum Arabic]. Gummisyrup.

Take of Mucilage of Gum Arabic *one part*, . . . 1
Simple Syrup *three parts*. 3

Mix them.

The Syrup is nearly colorless

Syrupus Ipecacuanhæ.

[SYRUP OF IPECACUANHA]. Ipecacuanhasyrup.

Take of Ipecacuanha, bruised, *one part*, ... 1
Diluted Alcohol *five parts*, ... 5
Distilled Water *thirty-six parts*, ... 36
and digest for twenty-four hours in a closed vessel.
Dissolve in *forty parts* 40
of the filtered liquid,
White Sugar *sixty-six parts*, ... 66
so as to form a syrup.

The Syrup has a yellowish color. *One hundred parts* correspond to *one part* of Ipecacuanha.

Syrupus Liquiritiæ.

[SYRUP OF LIQUORICE]. Süssholzsyrup.

Syrupus Glycyrrhizæ.

Take of Peeled Liquorice Root, cut, *four parts*, . . . 4
Common Water *eighteen parts*, ... 18
and macerate for one night. Bring the expresed and filtered liquid to the boiling point, then evaporate, by means of a steam-bath, so that there shall remain, after cooling and filtration, *seven parts*, ... 7
in which dissolve
White Sugar, ... 12
Clarified Honey, each, *twelve parts*. 12

Syrup of Liquorice has a yellowish-brown color.

Syrupus Mannæ.

[SYRUP OF MANNA]. Mannasyrup.

Take of Common Manna *three parts*. 3
Dissolve it in
Distilled Water *twelve parts*. 12
To the filtered liquid add of
White Sugar *sixteen parts*. 16

Heat them to the boiling-point, so as to form a syrup.

Syrup of Manna has a yellowish color.

Syrupus Menthæ crispæ.

[SYRUP OF CURLED-MINT]. Krauzeminzsyrup.

It is prepared from Curled-Mint Leaves, like Syrup of Chamomile.

It has a greenish-brown color.

Syrupus Menthæ piperitæ.

[SYRUP OF PEPPERMINT]. Pfefferminzsyrup.

It is prepared from Peppermint, like Syrup of Chamomile.
It has a greenish-brown color.

Syrupus opiatus.

[SYRUP OF OPIUM]. Opiumsyrup.

Take of Extract of Opium *one part*. 1

Dissolve it in a small quantity of Genuine White Wine, and mix with

Simple Syrup *one thousand parts*. . . . 1000

Syrupus Papaveris.

[SYRUP OF POPPIES]. Beruhigungssaft.

Syrupus Capitum Papaveris. Syrupus Diacodii.

Take of Poppy Heads, deprived of seeds and cut, . . . 3
St. John's Bread, cut, each, *three parts*, . . . 3
Peeled Liquorice Root, cut, *two parts*. . . . 2

Pour upon them

Hot Common Water *fifty parts*, ... 50

digest for two hours, in a steam-bath, and express. Evaporate the filtered liquid, by means of the steam-bath, so that there shall remain, after filtration, *fifteen parts*, . 15
in which dissolve

White Sugar *twenty-five parts*. 25

Syrup of Poppies has a yellowish-brown color.

Syrupus Rhamni catharticæ.

[SYRUP OF BUCKTHORN]. Kreuzdornbeerensyrup.

Syrupus Spinæ cervinæ. Syrupus domesticus.

It is prepared from fresh Buckthorn Berries, like Syrup of Cherries.

It has a violet color.

Syrupus Rhei.

[SYRUP OF RHUBARB]. Rhabarbersaft.

Take of Rhubarb, cut, *twelve parts*, ... 12
Cassia Bark, bruised, *three parts*, ... 3
Pure Carbonate of Potassium *one part*, . . 1
Distilled Water *one hundred parts*. . . . 100
Macerate for one night. Dissolve in *eighty parts* . 80
of the strained and filtered liquid,
White Sugar *one hundred and forty-four parts*. . 144
Syrup of Rhubarb has a brownish-red color.

Syrupus Rhœados.

[SYRUP OF RED POPPIES]. Klatschrosensaft.

Take of fresh Red Poppies *twelve parts*, ... 12
Hot Common Water *twenty parts*, ... 20
macerate for a night. Express gently and strain.
Dissolve in *twenty parts* 20
of the liquid,
White Sugar *thirty-six parts*, ... 36
so as to form a syrup.
The Syrup has a deep-red color.

Syrupus Rubi Idæi.

[SYRUP OF RASPBERRY]. Himbeersyrup.

The Juice of Raspberry is prepared from the bruised fresh raspberries, like the Juice of Cherries.

Dissolve in *five parts* 5
of Raspberry Juice, thus prepared,
White Sugar *nine parts*, ... 9
so as to form a syrup.

Syrup of Raspberry has a red color. The red color of the Syrup must not change to yellow on the addition of half its volume of nitric acid.

Syrupus Sarsaparillæ compositus.

[COMPOUND SYRUP OF SARSAPARILLA]. Zusammengesetzter Sassaparillsyrup.

Take of Sarsaparilla, cut, *twenty-four parts*, ... 24
Guaiacum Wood, rasped, ... 16
Sassafras Wood, cut, ... 16
China Root, cut, each, *sixteen parts*, . . . 16
Brown [Pale] Cinchona, bruised, *eight parts*, . 8
Anise, bruised, *three parts*. 3
Pour upon them
Hot Common Water *two hundred and fifty parts*. 250
Let them digest gently for a few hours, then express. Evaporate the filtered liquid, in a steam-bath, so that there shall remain *eighty parts*, ... 80
in which dissolve,
White Sugar *one hundred and thirty parts*, . 130
so as to form a syrup.

The Syrup has a brown color.

Syrupus Senegæ.

[SYRUP OF SENEKA]. Senegasyrup.

Take of Seneka Root, cut, *two parts*, ... 2
Distilled Water *twenty-two parts*, ... 22
Alcohol *three parts*, ... 3
macerate for two days, then express and filter.
Dissolve in *twenty-two parts* 22
of the filtered liquid,
White Sugar *thirty-six parts*, ... 36
so as to form a syrup.
Syrup of Seneka has a yellowish color.

Syrupus Sennæ cum Manna.

[SYRUP OF SENNA WITH MANNA]. Sennasyrup mit Manna.

Take of Senna, cut, *ten parts*, ... 10
Fennel Seeds, bruised, *one part*, ... 1
Hot Common Water *fifty parts*. 50
Set them aside for a few hours, shaking occasionally, then express. Dissolve in the liquid
Common Manna *fifteen parts*, ... 15
and strain.
Allow the liquid to settle, and dissolve in *fifty-five parts* 55
of the clear portion,
White Sugar *fifty parts*, ... 50
so as to form a syrup.
The Syrup has a brown color.

Syrupus Simplex.

[SIMPLE SYRUP]. Weisser Syrup.

Syrupus Sacchari. Syrupus albus.

Take of White Sugar *eighteen parts*, ... 18
Dissolve it in
Distilled Water *ten parts*, ... 10
so as to form a syrup.
Simple Syrup is colorless.

Syrupus Succi Citri.

[SYRUP OF LEMON]. Citronensaftsyrup.

Take of Lemons *a desired number.*
Express them, and dissolve in *ten parts* 10
of the expressed, clarified and filtered juice,
White Sugar *eighteen parts,* 18
so as to form a syrup.

Syrup of Lemon has a yellowish color.

Tartarus boraxatus.

[BORO-TARTRATE OF POTASSIUM]. Boraxweinstein.

Kali tartaricum boraxatum. Cremor Tartari solubilis.

Take of Borax *two parts*.. 2
Introduce it into a porcelain vessel, dissolve it in
Distilled Water *twenty parts,* 20
and add of
Bitartrate of Potassium *five parts*. . . . 5

Let the mixture remain in a steam-bath, stirring frequently, until the Bitartrate of Potassium has dissolved. Evaporate the filtered liquid in the steam-bath to a tough mass, which becomes friable on cooling. Draw out this mass into ribbons, and dry them with a gentle heat; then reduce them into powder, and introduce it immediately into a previously warmed vessel, which must be well closed.

A white powder, very deliquescent in the air, having a sour taste, and dissolving in an equal part of water.

The aqueous solution should not be affected by hydrosulphuric acid, or hydrosulphate of ammonium.

Tartarus depuratus.

[BITARTRATE OF POTASSIUM]. Weinstein.

[Cream of Tartar. Acid Tartrate of Potassium]. Kali bitartaricum purum. Cremor Tartari. Crystalli Tartari.

In white, hard, irregularly-formed crystals, or in a white crystalline powder, of an acidulous taste; soluble in one hundred and eighty parts of cold, and in from eighteen to twenty parts of boiling water; insoluble in alcohol. Solution of carbonate of potassium, and diluted solution of caustic potassa, dissolve it entirely, the former solution with effervescence.

Cream of tartar should not be colored when hydrosulphuric acid is poured upon it. The aqueous solution, mixed with a little nitric acid, should not be rendered turbid by chloride of barium, and only very slightly so by nitrate of silver. Dissolved in water of ammonia, the solution should not be altered by hydrosulphate of ammonium, nor precipitated by oxalate of ammonium.

Tartarus ferratus.

[FERRO-TARTRATE OF POTASSIUM]. Eisenweinstein.

Ferro-Kali tartaricum. In place of Globuli martiales.

Take of Iron Filings *one part*, ... 1
Bitartrate of Potassium, commercial, powdered, *five parts*. 5

Mix and convert them into a paste, with common water, in an earthenware vessel. Digest with frequent stirring, adding water as much as is lost by evaporation, until a uniform black mass is obtained, and a sample of it is found to be almost wholly soluble in water, forming a greenish-black solution. Then dry the mass in a moderately warm place, and reduce it to powder.

It forms a dirty-greenish powder, which assumes a brown color by age. When heated it diffuses a peculiar odor, burns and leaves a residue, which has a strongly aklaline reaction. It dissolves almost wholly in sixteen parts of cold water, forming a blackish-green solution.

Tartarus natronatus.

[TARTRATE OF POTASSIUM AND SODIUM]. Seignettesalz.

[Rochelle Salt. Seignette Salt. Tartarated Soda].

Natro-Kali tartaricum. Sal polychrestum Seignetti.

In rather large, transparent, rhombic prismatic crystals, soluble in one part and a half of cold, and one-third part of boiling water.

The aqueous solution should not be altered by hydrosulphuric acid, hydrosulphate of ammonium or oxalate of ammonium; and, after the addition of a little nitric acid, chloride of barium should produce no cloudiness, and nitrate of silver but a slight one.

Tartarus stibiatus.

[TARTRATE OF ANTIMONY AND POTASSIUM]. Brechweinstein.

[Tartar Emetic. Tartarated Antimony].

Tartarus emeticus. Stibio-Kali tartaricum.

A very white crystalline powder, of a feebly sweetish nauseous metallic taste. It chars upon the application of heat; is soluble in fifteen parts of cold, and in two parts of boiling water; insoluble in alcohol. It slightly reddens blue test paper.

The aqueous solution, to which has been added a little tartaric acid, should not be rendered turbid by chloride of barium, nitrate of silver or oxalate of ammonium; and when mixed with acetic acid, should not be altered by ferrocyanide of potassium. When dissolved in hydrochloric acid, the addition of a small quantity of protochloride of tin should produce no brown coloration in the solution on warming it.

It should be *cautiously* preserved.

Terebinthina.

[TURPENTINE]. Terpenthin.

[European Turpentine]. Terebinthina communis.

Pinus Pinaster *Aiton*, and of other species of Pinus.

A balsam of a variable consistence. It is somewhat granular, tenacious, opaque, and flows with difficulty. Its color is whitish, yellowish, or brownish-yellow. It has a strong, peculiar odor, and a bitter taste.

Terebinthina laricina.

[VENICE TURPENTINE]. Lärchenterpenthin.

Terebinthina Laricis. Terebinthina Veneta.

Larix decidua *Miller*.

A balsam which is generally transparent, sometimes slightly cloudy; it is homogenous, tenacious, and of a somewhat thick consistence. It has a yellowish or greenish-yellow color, a balsamic odor, and a bitter taste.

Tincturæ.

[TINCTURES]. Tincturen.

Tinctures are prepared, when no other process is given, in the following manner: The ingredients are coarsely powdered, or finely cut, and the extracting liquid (menstruum) is poured upon them in a bottle, which should be only partly filled. Maceration or digestion, according to directions, is then carried on for eight days, in a shady place, shaking frequently each day.

Maceration is conducted in well-closed vessels, at a temperature of between 15° and 20° C.; digestion in vessels only half filled and closed with a piece of bladder, pierced with a needle, at a heat of between 35° and 40° C.

When the maceration or digestion is completed, the cold liquid is poured off, and the residue expressed, which is done, if necessary, by means of a press. The liquid is then allowed to stand for twenty-four hours in the place where the tincture is intended to be kept, and is filtered in the same place, the funnel being covered with a glass plate. The small quantity of liquid lost by evaporation, during the preparation of the tincture, is not allowed to be replaced.

The tinctures should be clear, free from sediment, and possess the peculiar odor of the substances from which they are prepared.

They should be preserved in well-closed vessels, in a shady place, which has a temperature of about 15° C.

Tinctura Absinthii.

[TINCTURE OF WORMWOOD]. Wermuthtinktur.

Take of Wormwood *one part*, ... 1
Diluted Alcohol *five parts*. 5

Prepare the tincture by digestion.

Tincture of Wormwood has a brownish-green color.

Tinctura Aconiti.

[TINCTURE OF ACONITE ROOT]. Eisenhuttinktur.

Take of Aconite Root, bruised, *one part*, ... 1
Diluted Alcohol *ten parts*. 10

Prepare the tincture by digestion.

The Tincture has a yellowish-brown color.

It should be *cautiously* preserved.

Tinctura Aloës.

[TINCTURE OF ALOES]. Aloëtinktur.

Take of Aloes *one part*, ... 1
Alcohol *five parts*. 5

The tincture is prepared by digestion.

Tincture of Aloes has a blackish-brown color.

Tincture Aloës composita.

[COMPOUND TINCTURE OF ALOES]. Zusammengesetzte Aloëtinktur.

[***Swedish Bitters***]. ***In place of Elixir ad longam vitam.***

Take of Aloes *nine parts*, ... 9
Gentian Root, ... 1
Rhubarb, ... 1
Zedoary Root, ... 1
Saffron, ... 1
Larch Agaric, each, *one part*. 1

Cut and bruise the ingredients, and pour upon them
Diluted Alcohol *two hundred parts*, ... 200
and prepare the tincture by digestion.

Compound Tincture of Aloes has a reddish-brown color.

Tinctura amara.

[BITTER TINCTURE]. Bittere Tinktur.

Take of Orange Berries, ... 2
European Centaury, ... 2
Gentian Root, each, *two parts*, ... 2
Zedoary Root *one part*. 1

Cut the ingredients, and pour upon them
Diluted Alcohol *thirty-five parts*, ... 35
and prepare the tincture by digestion.

Bitter Tincture has a brown color with a faint greenish tint.

Tinctura Arnicæ.

[TINCTURE OF ARNICA]. Arnikatinktur.

It is prepared from Arnica Flowers, like Tincture of Aconite Root.

Tincture of Arnica has a brownish-yellow color.

Tinctura aromatica.

[AROMATIC TINCTURE]. Aromatische Tinktur.

Take of	Cassia Bark, coarsely powdered, *four parts*, .	4
	Small Cardamom, ...	1
	Cloves, ...	1
	Galangal Root, ...	1
	Ginger, each, coarsely powdered, *one part*, .	1
	Diluted Alcohol *fifty parts*.	50

Prepare the tincture by digestion.

Aromatic Tincture has a brownish-red color.

Tinctura aromatica acida.

[ACID AROMATIC TINCTURE]. Saure aromatische Tinktur.

In place of Elixir Vitrioli Mynsichti. [***Elixir of Vitriol***].

It is prepared like Aromatic Tincture, except to the
Diluted Alcohol *fifty parts*, ... 50
is added, before digestion,
Pure Sulphuric Acid *two parts*. 2

The Tincture has a brownish-red color.

Tinctura Asæ fœtidæ.

[TINCTURE OF ASSAFETIDA]. Stinkasanttinktur.

It is prepared from Assafetida, like Tincture of Aloes.
Tincture of Assafetida has a yellowish red-brown color.

Tinctura Aurantii Corticis.

[TINCTURE OF ORANGE PEEL]. Pomeranzenschalentinktur.

It is prepared from Orange Peel, like Tincture of Wormwood.

Tincture of Orange Peel has a brownish color.

Tincturæ Belladonnæ.

[TINCTURE OF BELLADONNA]. Belladonnatinktur.

Take of the fresh Leaves of Belladonna, with the flowering branches, *five parts*. 5
Having bruised them in a stone mortar, pour on Alcohol *six parts*, ... 6
and prepare the tincture by maceration.

Tincture of Belladonna has a brownish-green color.
It should be *cautiously* preserved.

Tinctura Benzoës.

[TINCTURE OF BENZOIN]. Benzoëtinktur.

It is prepared from Benzoin, like Tincture of Aloes.
Tincture of Benzoin has a yellowish brown-red color.

Tinctura Calami.

[TINCTURE OF CALAMUS]. Kalmustinktur.

It is prepared, by maceration, from Calamus Root, like Tincture of Wormwood.

Tincture of Calamus has a brownish-yellow color.

Tinctura Cannabis Indicæ.

[TINCTURE OF INDIAN HEMP]. Indischhanftinktur.

Take of Extract of Indian Hemp *one part*. . . . 1
Dissolve it in
Alcohol *nineteen parts*, ... 19
and filter.

Tincture of Indian Hemp has a greenish color.

It should be *cautiously* preserved.

Tinctura Cantharidum.

[TINCTURE OF CANTHARIDES]. Spanischfliegentinktur.

Take of Cantharides, coarsely powdered, *one part*, . 1
Alcohol *ten parts*, ... 10
and prepare the tincture by maceration.

Tincture of Cantharides has a yellowish-green color.

It should be *cautiously* preserved.

Tinctura Capsici.

[TINCTURE OF CAPSICUM]. Spanischpfeffertinktur.

It is prepared from finely-cut Capsicum, like Tincture of Cantharides.

Tincture of Capsicum has a brownish orange-yellow color.

It should be *cautiously* preserved.

Tinctura Cascarillæ.

[TINCTURE OF CASCARILLA]. Kaskarilltinktur.

It is prepared from Cascarilla Bark, like Tincture of Wormwood.

Tincture of Cascarilla has a reddish-brown color.

Tinctura Castorei Canadensis.

[Tincture of Canada Castor]. Tinktur aus Canadischem Bibergeil.

It is prepared from Canada Castor, like Tincture of Cantharides.

The Tincture has a dark-brown color.

Tinctura Castorei Sibirici.

[Tincture of Siberian Castor]. Tinktur aus Sibirischem Bibergeil.

It is prepared from Siberian Castor, like Tincture of Cantharides.

The Tincture has a reddish-brown color.

Tinctura Catechu.

[Tincture of Catechu]. Katechutinktur.

It is prepared from Catechu, like Tincture of Wormwood.

Tincture of Catechu has a dark-brown color.

Tinctura Chinæ.

[Tincture of Cinchona]. Chinatinktur.

It is prepared from Brown [Pale] Cinchona, like Tincture of Wormwood.

Tincture of Cinchona has a reddish-brown color.

Tinctura Chinæ composita.

[COMPOUND TINCTURE OF CINCHONA]. Zusammengesetzte Chinatinktur.

Elixir roborans Whyttii.

Take of Brown [Pale] Cinchona *six parts*,	. . .	6
Orange Peel,	. . . .	2
Gentian Root, each, *two parts*,	. . . .	2
Cassia Bark *one part*.	. . . . . .	1

Having cut and bruised the ingredients, pour upon them

Diluted Alcohol *fifty parts*,	. . . . .	50

and prepare a tincture by digestion.

The Tincture has a reddish-brown color.

Tinctura Chinoidini.

[TINCTURE OF QUINOIDIN]. Chinoidintinktur.

Take of Quinoidin *two parts*.	. . . .	2

Dissolve it in

Alcohol *seventeen parts*,	. . . . . .	17
Pure Hydrochloric Acid *one part*,	. . . .	1

and filter.

The Tincture has a brown color.

Tinctura Cinnamomi.

[TINCTURE OF CINNAMON]. Zimmttinktur.

It is prepared from Cassia Bark, like Tincture of Wormwood.

The Tincture has a reddish-brown color.

Tinctura Colchici.

[TINCTURE OF COLCHICUM.] Zeitlosentinktur.

[Tincture of Colchicum Seed]. Tinctura Seminis Colchici.

It is prepared from well bruised Colchicum Seeds, like Tincture of Aconite Root.

Tincture of Colchicum has a yellow color.

It should be *cautiously* preserved.

Tinctura Colocynthidis.

[TINCTURE OF COLOCYNTH]. Koloquintentinktur.

It is prepared from Colocynth, freed from the seeds, like Tincture of Cantharides.

The Tincture has a yellow color.

It should be *cautiously* preserved.

Tinctura Croci.

[TINCTURE OF SAFFRON]. Safrantinktur.

It is prepared by maceration from Saffron, like Tincture of Aconite Root.

Tincture of Saffron has a dark orange-yellow color.

Tinctura Digitalis.

[TINCTURE OF DIGITALIS]. Fingerhuttinktur.

It is prepared from the fresh Leaves of Digitalis, like Tincture of Belladonna.

Tincture of Digitalis has a brownish-green color.

It should be *cautiously* preserved.

Tinctura Digitalis æetherea.

[ETHEREAL TINCTURE OF DIGITALIS]. Aetherische Fingerhuttinktur.

Take of Digitalis Leaves *one part*, ... 1
Spirit of Ether *ten parts*. 10

Prepare the tincture by maceration.

It has a dark-green color.

It should be *cautiously* preserved.

Tinctura Euphorbii.

[TINCTURE OF EUPHORBIUM]. Euphorbiumtinktur.

It is prepared by digestion from Euphorbium, like Tincture of Cantharides.

Tincture of Euphorbium has a reddish-yellow color.

It should be *cautiously* preserved.

Tinctura Ferri acetici ætherea.

[ETHEREAL TINCTURE OF ACETATE OF IRON]. Aetherische essigsaure Eisentinktur.

Take of Solution of Acetate of Iron *nine parts*, . . 9
Alcohol *two parts*, ... 2
Acetic Ether *one part*. 1

Mix them.

The Tincture has a brown color.

It contains six per cent. of Iron.

Tinctura Ferri chlorati.

[TINCTURE OF PROTOCHLORIDE OF IRON]. Chloreisentinktur.

Take of Protochloride of Iron, recently prepared, *twenty-five parts*. 25

Dissolve it in
Diluted Alcohol *two hundred and twenty-five parts*, ... 225

add of
Pure Hydrochloric Acid *one part*, ... 1

mix and filter.

The Tincture is clear, with a yellowish-green color.

It should be preserved in rather small, well-closed bottles.

Tinctura Ferri chlorati ætherea.

[ETHEREAL TINCTURE OF CHLORIDE OF IRON]. Aetherische Chloreisentinktur.

Spiritus Ferri chlorati æthereus. Liquor anodynus martiatus. In place of Tinctura tonico-nervina Bestuscheffii.

Take of Solution of Sesquichloride of Iron *one part*, . 1
Spirit of Ether *fourteen parts*. 14

Mix and expose the liquid to the rays of the sun in well-closed, cylindrical bottles, until the brown-yellow color has wholly disappeared; then set aside in a shady place, opening the bottles occasionally, until the mixture has assumed a yellowish or brownish-yellow color.

The Tincture is clear, with a yellowish or brownish-yellow color. It contains one per cent. of Iron.

It should be preserved in well-closed glass-stoppered bottles.

Tinctura Ferri pomata.

[TINCTURE OF FERRATED EXTRACT OF APPLES]. Aepfelsaure Eisentinktur.

Take of Ferrated Extract of Apples *one part*. . . 1
Dissolve it in
Spirituous Cinnamon Water *nine parts*, . . 9
and filter.

The Tincture has a brownish-black color.

Tinctura Formicarum.

[TINCTURE OF ANTS]. Ameisentinktur.

Take of Ants, freshly collected, freed from impurities, and bruised, *two parts*, ... 2
Alcohol *three parts*. 3

Prepare the Tincture by digestion.

It has a brown color.

Tinctura Gallarum.

[TINCTURE OF NUTGALL]. Galläpfeltinktur.

Take of Nutgall, coarsely powdered, *one part*, . . 1
Diluted Alcohol *five parts*. 5

The tincture is prepared by digestion.

Tincture of Nutgall has a yellowish-brown color.

Tinctura Gentianæ.

[TINCTURE OF GENTIAN]. Enziantinktur.

It is prepared from Gentian Root, like Tincture of Wormwood.

Tincture of Gentian has a brownish-red color.

Tinctura Guajaci.

[TINCTURE OF GUAIAC]. Guajaktinktur.

It is prepared from Guaiac, like Tincture of Aloes.

Tincture of Guaiac has a dark red-brown color.

Tinctura Guajaci ammoniata.

[AMMONIATED TINCTURE OF GUAIAC]. Ammoniakalische Guajaktinktur.

Take of Guaiac, powered, *three parts*, ... 3
Alcohol *ten parts*, ... 10
Water of Ammonia *five parts*. 5

Prepare the tincture by maceration.

It has a greenish-brown color.

Tinctura Hellebori viridis.

[TINCTURE OF EUROPEAN GREEN HELLEBORE]. Nieswurzeltinktur.

It is prepared from European Green Hellebore, like Tincture of Aconite Root.

The Tincture has a yellowish-brown color.

It should be *cautiously* preserved.

Tinctura Iodi.

[TINCTURE OF IODINE]. Jodtinktur.

Take of Iodine *one part*. 1

Dissolve it in

Alcohol *ten parts*. 10

Pour off the clear liquid from the sediment.

Tincture of Iodine has a dark red-brown color.

It should be *cautiously* preserved in a glass-stoppered bottle.

Tinctura Iodi decolorata.

[COLORLESS TINCTURE OF IODINE]. Farblose Jodtinktur.

Take of Iodine, ... 10

Hyposulphite of Sodium, ... 10

Distilled Water, each, *ten parts*. . . . 10

Digest at a gentle heat, and shake occasionally, until solution is effected; then add of

Spirit of Ammonia *sixteen parts*, . . . 16

shake for a few minutes, and add of

Alcohol *seventy-five parts*. 75

Let the mixture stand for three days in a cool place, then filter.

It forms a clear, colorless liquid, having a peculiar and feebly ammoniacal odor, and a specific gravity of between 0.940 and 0.945.

It should be *cautiously* preserved.

Tinctura Ipecacuanhæ.

[TINCTURE OF IPECACUANHA]. Ipecacuanhatinktur.

It is prepared from Ipecacuanha, like Tincture of Aconite Root.

The Tincture has a reddish-brown color.

It should be *cautiously* preserved.

Tinctura Kino.

[TINCTURE OF KINO]. Kinotinktur.

Take of Kino, powdered, *one part*, ... 1
Alcohol *five parts*. 5

Prepare the tincture by maceration.

Tincture of Kino has a dark red-brown color.

Tinctura Lobeliæ.

[TINCTURE OF LOBELIA]. Lobeliatinktur.

It is prepared from Lobelia, like Tincture of Aconite Root.

The Tincture has a brownish-green color.

Tinctura Macidis.

[TINCTURE OF MACE]. Macistinktur.

It is prepared from Mace, like Tincture of Aloes.

Tincture of Mace has a reddish-yellow color.

Tinctura Moschi.

[TINCTURE OF MUSK]. Moschustinktur.

Take of Musk *one part*. 1
Triturate it intimately in a mortar with
Distilled Water *twenty-five parts*, ... 25
add of
Diluted Alcohol *twenty-five parts;* 25
then prepare the tincture by maceration.

Tincture of Musk has a reddish-brown color.

Tinctura Myrrhæ.

[TINCTURE OF MYRRH]. Myrrhentinktur.

It is prepared from coarsely powdered Myrrh, like Tincture of Aloes.

Tincture of Myrrh has a brown reddish-yellow color.

Tinctura Opii benzoica.

[CAMPHORATED TINCTURE OF OPIUM]. Benzoësäurehaltige Opiumtinktur.

[*Paregoric Elixir*]. *Elixir paregoricum.*

Take of Opium, powdered, *one part*, ...	1
Sublimed Benzoic Acid *four parts*, . . .	4
Camphor, ...	2
Oil of Anise, each, *two parts*, ...	2
Diluted Alcohol *one hundred and ninety-two parts*.	192

Prepare the tincture by digestion.

It has a yellow-brownish color.

It should be *cautiously* preserved.

REMARK.—*Two hundred parts* 200
of the Tincture contain the soluble portion of *one part* 1
of powdered Opium.

Tinctura Opii crocata.

[TINCTURE OF OPIUM AND SAFFRON]. Safranhaltige Opiumtinktur.

[*Sydenham's Laudanum*]. *Laudanum liquidum Sydenhami.*

Take of Opium, powdered, *sixteen parts*, ...	16
Saffron *six parts*, ...	6
Cloves, powdered, ...	1
Cassia Bark, powdered, each, *one part*, . .	1
Sherry Wine, *one hundred and fifty-two parts*. .	152

Prepare the tincture by digestion.

It has a dark saffron-brownish color, and a specific gravity of from 1.018 to 1.022.

It should be *cautiously* preserved.

REMARK.—*Ten parts* 10
of the Tincture contain the soluble portion of *one part* 1
of powdered Opium.

Tinctura Opii simplex.

[Tincture of Opium]. Einfache Opiumtinktur.

[*Laudanum*]. *Tinctura Thebaica. Tinctura Meconii.*

Take of Opium, powdered, *four parts*, ...	4
Diluted Alcohol, ...	19
Distilled Water, each, *nineteen parts*. . .	19

Prepare the tincture by digestion.

It has a dark reddish-brown color, and a specific gravity of from 0.978 to 0.982.

It should be *cautiously* preserved.

Remark.—*Ten parts*	10
of the Tincture contain the soluble portion of *one part*	1
of powdered Opium.	

Tinctura Pimpinellæ.

[Tincture of Pimpinel]. Pimpinelltinktur.

It is prepared from *Radix Pimpinella*, like Tincture of Wormwood.

The Tincture has a brownish-yellow color.

Tinctura Pini composita.

[Tincture of Woods]. Holztinktur.

Tinctura Lignorum.

Take of young Pine-shoots (*Turiones Pini*), cut, *three parts*, ...	3
Guaiac Wood, rasped, *two parts*, ...	2
Sassafras Wood, rasped, ...	1
Juniper Berries, bruised, each, *one part*, . . .	1
Diluted Alcohol *thirty-six parts*.	36

Prepare the tincture by digestion.

It has a brown color.

Tinctura Ratanhæ.

[TINCTURE OF RHATANY]. Ratanhatinktur.

It is prepared from Rhatany Root, like Tincture of Wormwood.

Tincture of Rhatany has a dark red-brown color.

Tinctura Resinæ Jalapæ.

[TINCTURE OF RESIN OF JALAP]. Jalapenharztinktur.

It is prepared from Resin of Jalap, like Tincture of Cantharides.

The Tincture has a brownish color.

It should be *cautiously* preserved.

Tinctura Rhei aquosa.

[AQUEOUS TINCTURE OF RHUBARB]. Wässrige Rhabarbertinktur.

Take of Rhubarb, cut, *one hundred parts*, ... 100
Borax, powdered, ... 10
Pure Carbonate of Potassium, each, *ten parts*. . 10
Pour upon them
Boiling Distilled Water *eight hundred and fifty parts*, ... 850
set aside for a quarter of an hour, then add of
Alcohol *one hundred parts*, ... 100
mix, and set aside again for one hour and a quarter.
Express gently, and to the filtered liquid add of
Cinnamon Water *one hundred and fifty parts*. . 150

The Tincture is clear, with a red-brown color, and an odor of Rhubarb.

Tinctura Rhei vinosa.

[VINOUS TINCTURE OF RHUBARB]. Weinige Rhabarbertinktur.

In place of Tinctura Rhei Darelii.

Take of	Rhubarb, finely cut, *eight parts,* . . .	8
	Orange Peel, cut, *two parts,*	2
	Small Cardamoms, powdered, *one part,* . .	1
	Sherry Wine *one hundred parts.*	100

Prepare the tincture by digestion, filter, and dissolve in it

White Sugar, powdered, *twelve parts.* . .	12

The Tincture has a yellowish-brown color.

Tinctura Scillæ.

[TINCTURE OF SQUILL]. Meerzwiebeltinktur.

It is prepared from dried Squill, like Tincture of Wormwood.

Tincture of Squill has a yellow color.

Tinctura Scillæ kalina.

[ALKALINE TINCTURE OF SQUILL]. Kalihaltige Meerzwiebeltinktur.

Take of	Squill, dried, *eight parts,*	8
	Caustic Potassa *one part,*	1
	Diluted Alcohol *fifty parts.*	50

Prepare the tincture by maceration.

It has a brownish color.

Tinctura Secalis cornuti.

[TINCTURE OF ERGOT]. Mutterkorntinktur.

It is prepared from powdered Ergot, like Tincture of Aconite Root.

Tincture of Ergot has a brownish-red color.

Tinctura Spilanthis composita.

[TINCTURE OF SPILANTHUS]. Paratinktur.

[*Paraguay Roux*].

Take of Spear-leaved Spilanthus, dried and coarsely powdered, ... 2
Pellitory Root, coarsely powdered, each, *two parts*, ... 2
Diluted Alcohol *ten parts*. 10

Prepare the tincture by digestion.

It has a greenish-brown color.

Tinctura Stramonii.

[TINCTURE OF STRAMONIUM]. Stechapfelsamentinktur.

It is prepared from coarsely powdered Stramonium Seeds, like Tincture of Aconite Root.

The Tincture has a brownish-yellow color.

It should be *cautiously* preserved.

Tinctura Strychni.

[TINCTURE OF NUX VOMICA]. Krähenaugentinktur.

Strychnostinktur.

It is prepared from Nux Vomica, like Tincture of Aconite Root.

Tincture of Nux Vomica has a yellow color.

It should be *cautiously* preserved.

Tinctura Strychni ætherea.

[ETHEREAL TINCTURE OF NUX VOMICA]. Aetherische Krähenaugentinktur.

Aetherische Strychnostinktur.

Take of Nux Vomica, coarsely powdered, *one part*, . 1
Spirit of Ether *ten parts*. 10

Prepare the tincture by maceration.

It has a yellowish color.

It should be *cautiously* preserved.

Tinctura Thujæ.

[TINCTURE OF ARBOR VITÆ]. Lebensbaumtinktur.

Tinctura Thujæ occidentalis.

It is prepared from the fresh Leaves of Arbor Vitæ (*Thuja occidentalis*) like tincture of Belladonna.

The Tincture has a greenish-yellow color.

Tinctura Toxicodendri.

[TINCTURE OF POISON OAK]. Giftsumachtinktur.

It is prepared from the fresh Leaves of Poison Oak, like Tincture of Belladonna.

The Tincture has a yellowish-green color.

It should be *cautiously* preserved.

Tinctura Valerianæ.

[TINCTURE OF VALERIAN]. Baldriantinktur.

It is prepared from finely cut Valerian Root, like Tincture of Wormwood.

Tincture of Valerian has a brown color.

Tinctura Valerianæ ætherea.

[ETHEREAL TINCTURE OF VALERIAN]. Aetherische Baldriantinktur.

Take of Valerian Root, coarsely powdered, *one part*, . 1
Spirit of Ether *five parts*. 5

Prepare the tincture by maceration.

It has a yellow color which assumes a brownish tint by age.

Tinctura Vanillæ.

[TINCTURE OF VANILLA]. Vanillentinktur.

It is prepared by maceration from Vanilla, like Tincture of Wormwood.

Tincture of Vanilla has a reddish-brown color.

Tinctura Zingiberis.

[TINCTURE OF GINGER]. Ingwertinktur.

It is prepared from coarsely powdered Ginger, like Tincture of Wormwood.

Tragacantha.

[TRAGACANTH]. Traganth.

[Gum Dragon]. Gummi Tragacantha.

Astragalus Creticus *Lamark*, and of other species of Astragalus.

It occurs in thin, flat, roundish pieces, which are spirally twisted, or more or less tortuous; curved like a sickle, and traversed by semi-circular, concentric, striated elevations; or in thin, filiform, somewhat cochleate-twisted pieces, traversed by smaller concentric, striated elevations. Tragacanth is a tough, white, or yellowish-white, almost translucent, inodorous substance, horny, and difficult of pulverization. It swells up when macerated in cold water, and yields a thick mucilage with boiling water.

Trochisci.

[TROCHES]. Pastillen.

[Lozenges].

Troches are to be prepared by adding the whole amount of the intended medicinal substance to sugar, which has been previously moistened with diluted alcohol; or it is mixed with a cacao-mass, softened by heat. The mass is well worked, spread out by means of a roller, and then properly divided into troches, each containing a definite quantity of the medicinal substance. The amount of sugar or cacao-mass must be so regulated that each troche shall weigh one gramme.

Trochisci Ipecacuanhæ.

[TROCHES OF IPECACUANHA]. Brechwurzelpastillen.

Take of Ipecacuanha, bruised, *two parts*, . . . 2
Hot Common Water *ten parts*, ... 10
set aside, in a warm place, for several hours, then strain. Mix the filtered liquid with
White Sugar, powdered, *a sufficient quantity*
to make the mass amount to *four hundred parts*, . . 400
from which prepare troches, each weighing one gramme.

Each troche contains the soluble portion of five milligrammes (0.005) of Ipecacuanha.

Trochisci Magnesiæ ustæ.

[TROCHES OF MAGNESIA]. Magnesiapastillen.

They are prepared with Magnesia and Cacao-mass, so that each troche shall contain one decigramme (0.1) of Magnesia.

Trochisci Morphini acetici.

[TROCHES OF ACETATE OF MORPHIA]. Morphinpastillen.

They are prepared with Acetate of Morphia and White Sugar, so that each troche shall contain five milligrammes (0.005) of Acetate of Morphia.

Trochisci Natri bicarbonici.

[TROCHES OF BICARBONATE OF SODIUM]. Natronpastillen.

Take of White Sugar, powdered, *eighteen parts*, . . 18
Bicarbonate of Sodium, powdered, *two parts*. . 2

Mix, and with alcohol form a mass, which divide into troches, each weighing one gramme.

Trochisci Santonini.

[TROCHES OF SANTONIN]. Santoninpastillen.

They are prepared with Santonin and Cacao-mass of two degrees of strength, so that each troche of one kind shall contain five centigrammes (0.05), and each troche of the other kind twenty-five milligrammes (0.025) of Santonin. Each kind must be kept in a separate vessel.

Tubera Aconiti.

[ACONITE ROOT OR TUBER]. Eisenhutknollen.

Aconitum Napellus, *Linn.*

The roots (tubers) are conical, with the broad part at the top, where each is provided with the remains of a stem, or bud [of the incipient stem]. They are frequently united in pairs; in such cases they are of different age. When dry the roots are hard, from five to eight centimetres in length, two to three centimetres in thickness at their upper extremity. The root of the present (one) year's growth is heavy, compact, and whitish internally; that of the last (two) year's growth is light in weight, brownish internally, and often hollow. Roots of both ages are brown externally, furrowed, and somewhat marked with scars where the rootlets have been cut off. On the cross section of the root is seen the thick and dotted bark, separated from the wide (large) stellately circumscribed pith by the very thin, darker-colored, circular, stellated woody part, which is marked with seven or eight very prominent rays.

The roots of *Aconitum Cammarum* Jacquin, should be rejected. They are smaller than those of *Aconitum Napellus;* they are about two centimetres long, and about twelve millimetres thick at the top, and have an unequally stellated wood and pith, and are marked with but slightly prominent rays. The roots of *Aconitum Stœrkianum* Reichenbach, should also be rejected; a number of them are generally united. They are much larger, their wood and pith are not stellated, but obtuse- or roundish-angled.

The roots of the wild-growing plant should be collected; they must be *cautiously* preserved.

Tubera Jalapæ.

[JALAP]. Jalapenknollen.

[*Jalap Root or Tuber*]. *Radix Jalapæ.*

Convolvulus Purga *Wenderoth,* (**Ipomœa Purga** *Hayne*).

The tubers are globular, pear-shaped, or oblong, of various sizes, and are either entire or divided. They are compact and heavy; externally wrinkled, and of a brown color; covered in the depressions of the wrinkles with a blackish resin. Internally of a light-brown color, and marked with numerous darker-colored concentric zones, which contain shining resiniferous cells.

Jalap should be *cautiously* preserved. The powder should contain at least ten per cent. of resin.

Tubera Salep.

[SALEP]. Salep.

Radix Salep.

Orchis Morio *Linn*, and of other species of Orchis.

The tubers are irregularly ovate, or oblong, rarely palmate; from one to two and a half centimetres in length, somewhat translucent, of a horny consistence, and of a dirty-white or whitish light-brown color. Powdered Salep yields a mucilage with water.

Care should be taken that the tubers are not mixed with colchicum root.

Turiones Pini.

[YOUNG PINE-SHOOTS]. Fichtensprossen.

[*Pine Buds*]. *Gemmæ Pini.*

Pinus silvestris *Linn.*

Cylindrical shoots [of the branches], upwards of five centimetres in length; they are glutinous when fresh, owing to a resinous exudation. The axis is green, closely imbricated, with numerous narrow scarious, rusty-colored scales, each of which supports and incloses a small pair of rudimental leaves, which are surrounded by a transparent sheath. They have a strong balsamic-resinous odor, and a bitterish-resinous taste.

They should be collected in the beginning of spring, upon a clear day, quickly dried, and preserved in closed vessels, but not kept longer than a year.

Unguentum acre.

[ACRID OINTMENT]. Scharfe Salbe. Hufsalbe.

Take of Yellow Wax *fifteen parts*, ... 15
Resin *thirty parts*, ... 30
Turpentine *sixty parts*, ... 60
Lard *two hundred and fifty parts*. . . . 250

Melt them together, add of
Cantharides, in fine powder, *fifty parts*, . . 50
Euphorbium, in fine powder, *ten parts*, . . 10

and mix.

The Ointment has a greenish-brown color.

Unguentum arsenicale Hellmundi.

[HELLMUND'S ARSENICAL OINTMENT]. Hellmund'sche Arseniksalbe.

Take of Arsenical Powder of Côme *one part*, ... 1
Hellmund's Narcotic-balsamic Ointment *eight parts*. 8

Mix them very thoroughly.

The Ointment has a grayish-brown color.

It is prepared only when wanted for dispensing.

Unguentum basilicum.

[BASILICON OINTMENT]. Königssalbe.

Take of Common Olive Oil *six parts*, ... 6
Yellow Wax, ... 2
Resin, ... 2
Suet, each, *two parts*, ... 2
Turpentine *one part*. 1

Melt them with a gentle heat, and strain.

It has a yellowish-brown color.

Unguentum Belladonnæ.

[OINTMENT OF BELLADONNA]. Tollkirschensalbe.

Take of Extract of Belladonna *one part*, ... 1
Wax Ointment *nine parts*. 9

Mix them very thoroughly.

It is prepared only when wanted for dispensing.

Unguentum Cantharidum.

[CANTHARIDES OINTMENT]. Spanischfliegensalbe.

Unguentum irritans. In place of Unguentum ad Fonticulos.

Take of Cantharides, bruised, *one part*, ... 1
Provence Olive Oil *four parts*. 4

Digest them in a steam-bath for twelve hours.

Express when cold, filter and add of
Yellow Wax *two parts*, ... 2

Melt them with a gentle heat, and stir constantly while cooling.

A greenish Ointment.

Unguentum cereum.

[WAX OINTMENT]. Wachssalbe.

Take of Provence Olive Oil *five parts*, ... 5
Yellow Wax *two parts*. 2

Melt them by means of a steam-bath, and stir while cooling.
Wax Ointment has a yellow color.

Unguentum Cerussæ.

[OINTMENT OF WHITE LEAD]. Bleiweisssalbe.

[*Ointment of Carbonate of Lead*]. *Unguentum Plumbi subcarbonici. Unguentum Plumbi hydrico-carbonici. Unguentum album simplex.*

Take of Lard *two parts*, ... 2
White Lead, in very fine powder, *one part*. . 1

Mix them very thoroughly.
A very white Ointment.

Unguentum Cerussæ camphoratum.

[CAMPHORATED OINTMENT OF WHITE LEAD]. Bleiweisssalbe mit Kampfer.

Take of Camphor, powdered, *five parts*, ... 5
Ointment of White Lead *one hundred parts*. . 100

Mix very thoroughly.
A very white Ointment.

Unguentum Conii.

[CONIUM OINTMENT]. Schierlingssalbe.

Take of Extract of Conium *one part*, ... 1
Wax Ointment *nine parts*.. 9

Mix them very thoroughly.
The Ointment is prepared only when wanted for dispensing.

Unguentum diachylon Hebræ.

[HEBRA'S OINTMENT OF LEAD]. Hebra'sche Bleisalbe.

Take of Lead Plaster, ... 1
Flaxseed Oil, each, *one part*. 1
Mix them properly at a gentle heat.
It is prepared only when wanted for dispensing.

Unguentum Digitalis.

[OINTMENT OF DIGITALIS]. Fingerhutsalbe.

Take of Extract of Digitalis *one part*, ... 1
Wax Ointment *nine parts*. 9
Mix them very thoroughly.
It is prepared only when wanted for dispensing.

Unguentum Elemi.

[OINTMENT OF ELEMI]. Elemisalbe.

Balsamum Arcæi.

Take of Elemi,
Venice Turpentine,
Suet,
Lard, each, *equal parts*.
Melt them by means of a steam-bath, and strain.
Ointment of Elemi has a greenish-gray or yellowish color.

Unguentum flavum.

[YELLOW OINTMENT]. Altheesalbe.

In place of Unguentum Althææ. [***Marshmallow Ointment***].

Take of Turmeric, powdered, *ten parts*, ... 10
Lard *five hundred parts*. 500
Digest for half an hour, in a steam-bath, then add of
Yellow Wax, ... 30
Burgundy Pitch, each, *thirty parts*. . . . 30
Melt them together and strain.
The Ointment has a yellow color.

Unguentum Glycerini.

[Glycerin Ointment]. Glycerinsalbe.

Take of Wheat Starch *two parts*, ... 2
Triturate it with
Distilled Water *one part*, ... 1
and add of
Glycerin *ten parts*. 10

Heat them by means of a steam-bath, until they are converted into a translucent, uniform mass.

Unguentum Hydrargyri cinereum.

[Mercurial Ointment]. Graue Quecksilbersalbe.

Unguentum Neapolitanum.

Take of Purified Mercury *six parts*, ... 6
Old Mercurial Ointment *one part*. 1
Rub them sedulously together, until the globules cease to be visible; then mix with
Suet *four parts*, ... 4
Lard *eight parts*, ... 8
which were previously melted and allowed to cool.

Mercurial Ointment has a bluish-gray color. No globules of mercury can be detected in it by the naked eye.

Unguentum Hydrargyri præcipitati albi.

[Ointment of Ammoniated Mercury]. Weisse Quecksilbersalbe.

Unguentum Hydrargyri amidato-bichlorati.

Take of Ammoniated Mercury *one part*, ... 1
Lard *nine parts*. 9

Mix them very thoroughly.

A very white ointment.

It is prepared only when wanted for dispensing.

Unguentum Hydrargyri rubrum.

[OINTMENT OF RED OXIDE OF MERCURY]. Rothe Quecksilbersalbe.

Take of Red Oxide of Mercury *one part*, ... 1
Lard *nine parts*. 9

Mix them very thoroughly.

A red ointment.

It is prepared only when wanted for dispensing.

Unguentum Hyoscyami.

[OINTMENT OF HYOSCYAMUS]. Bilsenkrautsalbe.

Take of Extract of Hyoscyamus *one part*, ... 1
Wax Ointment *nine parts*. 9

Mix very thoroughly.

It is prepared only when wanted for dispensing.

Unguentum Kalii iodati.

[OINTMENT OF IODIDE OF POTASSIUM]. Jodkaliumsalbe.

Take of Iodide of Potassium *twenty parts*, ... 20
Hyposulphite of Sodium *one part*. 1

Dissolve, by rubbing them together, in
Distilled Water *fifteen parts*, ... 15

and mix with
Lard *one hundred and sixty-five parts*. . . 165

It forms a very white Ointment.

Unguentum leniens.

[COLD CREAM]. Cold-Cream.

Take of White Wax *four parts*, ... 4
Spermaceti *five parts*, ... 5
Expressed Oil of Almonds *thirty-two parts*. . 32

Melt them in a steam-bath, and when cool, while constantly stirring, gradually add of
Rose Water *sixteen parts*. 16

To each fifty grammes of the ointment mix
Oil of Rose *one drop*.

Cold Cream is a soft and very white ointment.

Unguentum Linariæ.

[OINTMENT OF TOAD-FLAX]. Leinkrautsalbe.

Take of Common Toad-Flax, cut, *two parts*. . . . 2
Sprinkle it with
Alcohol *one part*. 1
Let it stand for several hours in a warm place; then add of
Lard *ten parts*, ... 10
digest in a steam-bath until the alcohol is entirely dissipated, then express and strain.

The Ointment has a greenish color.

Unguentum Majoranæ.

[OINTMENT OF SWEET MARJORAM]. Meiransalbe.

It is prepared from Sweet Marjoram, like Ointment of Toad-Flax.

The Ointment has a green color.

Unguentum Mezerei.

[MEZEREON OINTMENT]. Seidelbastsalbe.

Take of Extract of Mezereon *one part*, ... 1
Wax Ointment *nine parts*. 9
Mix very thoroughly.

It is prepared only when wanted for dispensing.

Unguentum narcotico-balsamicum Hellmundi.

[HELLMUND'S NARCOTIC-BALSAMIC OINTMENT]. Hellmünd's narkotisch-balsamische Salbe.

Take of Acetate of Lead, very finely triturated, *ten parts*, 10
Extract of Conium *thirty parts*. . . . 30
Mix very thoroughly, and add of
Wax Ointment *two hundred and forty parts*, . 240
Balsam of Peru *thirty parts*, ... 30
Tincture of Opium and Saffron *five parts*. . 5
It forms a brownish Ointment.

Unguentum ophthalmicum.

[EYE-SALVE]. Augensalbe.

Take of Expressed Oil of Almonds *thirty parts*, . . 30
Yellow Wax *nineteen parts*. 19
Melt, and when cool add of
Red Oxide of Mercury *one part*, . . . 1
and mix.
It forms a reddish Ointment.

Unguentum ophthalmicum compositum.

[COMPOUND EYE-SALVE]. Zusammengesetzte rothe Augensalbe.

Unguentum ophthalmicum St. Yves.

Take of Lard *one hundred and forty parts*, . . . 140
Yellow Wax *twenty-four parts*, ... 24
Red Oxide of Mercury *fifteen parts*, . . . 15
Pure Oxide of Zinc *six parts*. 6
Mix, and add of
Camphor *five parts*, ... 5
previously dissolved in
Expressed Oil of Almonds *ten parts*. . . 10
It forms a yellowish-red Ointment.

Unguentum opiatum.

[OPIUM OINTMENT]. Opiumsalbe.

Take of Extract of Opium, ... 1
Distilled Water, each, *one part*. 1
Rub them together, and mix very thoroughly with
Wax Ointment *eighteen parts*. 18

The Ointment is prepared only when wanted for dispensing.

Unguentum oxygenatum.

[OXYGENATED OINTMENT]. Oxygenirte Salbe.

Take of Lard *fifty parts.* 50
Melt it in a porcelain vessel, and add of
Pure Nitric Acid *three parts.* 3

Heat them with a gentle heat, stirring constantly with a glass rod, until the mixture no longer reddens blue test-paper. Then pour the mass into paper capsules, and preserve the cold ointment in a closed vessel.

It has the consistence of a cerate, a yellowish color, and an odor as if it were rancid.

Unguentum Plumbi.

[OINTMENT OF SUBACETATE OF LEAD]. Bleisalbe.

Bleicerat.

Take of Yellow Wax *eight parts,* 8
Lard *twenty-nine parts.* 29

Melt them in a steam bath, and mix the partially cooled mass with
Solution of Subacetate of Lead *three parts,* . 3
and stir while cooling.

The Ointment has a yellowish color.

Unguentum Plumbi tannici.

[OINTMENT OF TANNATE OF LEAD]. Gerbsaure Bleisalbe.

Unguentum ad Decubitum.

Take of Oak Bark, cut, *sixteen parts,* 16
Distilled Water *eighty parts,* 80
digest for two hours in a steam-bath, and express.

To the strained liquid, while stirring constantly, add of,
Solution of Subacetate of Lead *eight parts.* . 8

Collect the resulting precipitate on a filter, and express it gently between folds of bibulous paper, so that the weight of the moist pulp shall be *eight parts,* . . 8
and mix it thoroughly with
Glycerin Ointment *five parts.* 5

It should be preserved in a cool place.

The Ointment has a reddish-brown color.

Unguentum Populi.

[Ointment of Poplar-buds]. Pappelsalbe.

Pappelpomade. Unguentum Populeum.

Take of Fresh Poplar-buds, bruised, *one part*, . . 1
Lard *two parts*. 2

Boil with a moderate heat, until all moisture is dissipated; then express and strain.

The Ointment has a greenish color.

Unguentum rosatum.

[Rose Ointment]. Rosensalbe.

Take of Lard *fifty parts*, ... 50
White Wax *ten parts*. 10

Melt by means of a steam-bath, and mix the partially cooled mass with

Rose Water *five parts*. 5

Rose Ointment is very white.

Unguentum Rosmarini compositum.

[Compound Rosemary Ointment]. Rosmarinsalbe.

[*Nerve Ointment*]. *Nervensalbe. Unguentum nervinum.*

Take of Lard *sixteen parts*, ... 16
Suet *eight parts*, ... 8
Yellow Wax, ... 2
Expressed Oil of Nutmeg, each, *two parts*. . 2

Melt by means of a steam-bath, and mix with the partially cooled mass

Oil of Rosemary, ... 1
Oil of Juniper Berries, each, *one part*. . . 1

The Ointment has a yellowish color.

Unguentum Sabinæ.

[Savine Ointment]. Sadebaumsalbe.

It is prepared from Extract of Savine, like Ointment of Belladonna.

It is prepared only when wanted for dispensing.

Unguentum Sulfuratum compositum.

[COMPOUND SULPHUR OINTMENT]. Zusammengesetzte Schwefelsalbe.

Take of Washed Sulphur, ...	1
Sulphate of Zinc, powdered, each, *one part*, .	1
Lard, *eight parts*.	8

Mix them.

The Ointment has a lemon-yellow color.

Unguentum Sulfuratum simplex.

[SULPHUR OINTMENT]. Schwefelsalbe.

Take of Washed Sulphur *one part*, ...	1
Lard *two parts*.	2

Mix them.

It is prepared only when wanted for dispensing.

Unguentum Tartari stibiati.

[ANTIMONIAL OINTMENT]. Pockensalbe.

[*Tartar Emetic Ointment*].
Unguentum stibiatum. Unguentum Stibio-Kali tartarici.

Take of Tartar Emetic *two parts*. 2

Rub it into a very fine powder, and mix thoroughly with

Lard *eight parts*. 8

It is prepared only when wanted for dispensing.

Unguentum Terebinthinæ.

[TURPENTINE OINTMENT]. Terpenthinsalbe.

Take of Turpentine, ...	1
Yellow Wax, each, *one part*.	1

Melt them with a gentle heat; mix with

Oil of Turpentine *one part*, ... 1

and stir while cooling.

Turpentine Ointment is somewhat soft, and has a yellowish color.

Unguentum Terebinthinæ compositum.

[COMPOUND TURPENTINE OINTMENT]. Zusammengesetzte Terpenthinsalbe.

Unguentum digestivum.

Take of Venice Turpentine *thirty-two parts*, . . . 32
Yolk of Egg *four parts*. 4
Stir them thoroughly together; then triturate with
Myrrh, powdered, ... 1
Aloes, powdered, each, *one part*, ... 1
Province Olive Oil *eight parts*. 8
The Ointment is soft, and has a tawny chestnut-brown color.

Unguentum Zinci.

[OINTMENT OF OXIDE OF ZINC]. Zinksalbe.

Take of Commercial Oxide of Zinc *one part*, ... 1
Rose Ointment *nine parts*. 9
Mix them very thoroughly.
The Ointment is very white.

Vanilla Saccharata.

[SACCHARATED VANILLA]. Vanillenzucker.

Take of Vanilla, finely cut, *one part*, ... 1
White Sugar *nine parts*. 9

Rub them together until they are mixed and converted into a whitish-gray powder.

It should be preserved in well-closed vessels.

Veratrinum.

[VERATRIA]. Veratrin.

A whitish powder, which readily conglomerates, and is sometimes crystalline. It has an alkaline reaction, and an acrid taste devoid of bitterness; but, even in the most minute quantity, producing violent sneezing. Scarcely soluble in cold or hot water; completely soluble in three parts of alcohol; also soluble in ether and diluted acids. It chars by a somewhat strong heat, and finally burns away at a red heat, leaving no residue. The acidulated aqueous solution, on the addition of solution of caustic potassa, yields a white precipitate, which is insoluble in an excess of the alkaline solution, but dissolves readily in alcohol, ether, or chloroform. Its alcoholic solution yields no precipitate with bichloride of platinum. Veratria forms, with concentrated hydrochloric acid, a cherry-red solution upon the application of heat. When mixed with sulphuric acid, it at first assumes a yellow color, which changes by a gentle heat to a scarlet, and finally to a violet color.

It should be very *cautiously* preserved.

Vinum.

[WINE*]. Wein.

Vitis vinifera ***Linn.***

For pharmaceutical purposes are used:

Genuine White Wine, *Vinum generosum album;*
Genuine Red Wine, *Vinum generosum rubrum;*
Sherry Wine, *Vinum Xerense.*

Vinum aromaticum.

[AROMATIC WINE]. Aromatischer Wein.

Take of Aromatic Spices *two parts,*	2
White Arquebusade *five parts,*	5
Genuine Red Wine *sixteen parts.*	16

Macerate for eight days, then express and filter.

Aromatic Wine is clear, with a reddish-brown color.

---

* Dr. Hager, in his Commentary on the *Phar. Germanica*, puts the percentage, by volume, of alcohol of the respective wines as follows: White and Red (French) Wines, from 10 to 12 per cent.; Sherry, from 16 to 20 per cent.; and Hock (Rhine Wine), from 8 to 10 per cent.

Vinum camphoratum.

[WINE OF CAMPHOR]. Kampferwein.

Take of	Camphor, powdered, ...	1
	Gum Arabic, finely powdered, each, *one part*. .	1

Mix by rubbing them intimately together, and, while constantly stirring, add of

	Genuine White Wine *forty-eight parts*. . .	48

It forms a whitish-turbid liquid.

Vinum Chinæ.

[WINE OF CINCHONA]. Chinawein.

Take of	Calisaya Bark *five parts*, ...	5
	Genuine Red Wine *one hundred parts*. . .	100

Macerate for eight days, then express and filter.

Wine of Cinchona has a red color, and a bitter taste.

Vinum Colchici.

[WINE OF COLCHICUM SEEDS]. Zeitlosensamenwein.

Take of	Colchicum Seeds, coarsely powdered, *one part*,	1
	Sherry Wine *ten parts*.	10

Macerate for eight days, then express and filter.

Wine of Colchicum Seeds has a yellowish-brown color.

It should be *cautiously* preserved in well-closed vessels.

Vinum Ipecacuanhæ.

[WINE OF IPECACUANHA]. Brechwurzelwein.

Take of	Ipecacuanha, coarsely powdered, *one part*, .	1
	Sherry Wine *ten parts*.	10

Macerate for eight days, then express and filter.

It is clear, with a yellowish-brown color.

It should be *cautiously* preserved in well-closed vessels.

Vinum Pepsini.

[WINE OF PEPSINE]. Pepsinwein.

Vinum pepticum. Essentia Pepsini.

Take the stomach of a hog, or the fourth stomach (abomasus) of an ox. Turn it inside out, and having freed it from the undigested matter, wash it with cold water; then strongly scrape off, by means of a bone spatula, the peptic mucus from the mucous membrane.

Mix carefully *one hundred parts* 100
of this Mucus with
Glycerin *fifty parts*, ... 50
which has been previously diluted with
Distilled Water *fifty parts*. 50

Introduce the mixture into a capacious flask; add of
Genuine White Wine *one thousand parts*, . . 1000
Pure Hydrochloric Acid *five parts*, . . . 5
and shake briskly. Then macerate, at a temperature not exceeding 20° C., for three days, shaking frequently, and finally filter.

Wine of Pepsine is a clear, yellowish liquid, and has a vinous, somewhat acidulous taste.

Vinum stibiatum.

[ANTIMONIAL WINE]. Brechwein.

Vinum emeticum. Vinum Stibio-Kali tartarici.

Take of Tartar Emetic *one part*. 1
Dissolve it in
Sherry Wine *two hundred and fifty parts*, . . 250
and filter.

Antimonial Wine is clear, with a brownish-yellow color.

It should be *cautiously* preserved in well-closed vessels.

Zincum aceticum.

[ACETATE OF ZINC]. Essigsaures Zinkoxyd.

In colorless, tabular, crystalline scales, soluble in three parts of cold, and in one part and a half of hot water, also soluble in alcohol. A slightly acidulous solution affords, with solution of caustic potassa, a white precipitate, which is redissolved in an excess of the alkaline solution, forming a liquid which yields again a white precipitate with hydrosulphuric acid.

The aqueous solution, on the addition of carbonate of ammonium, throws down a precipitate, which is entirely redissolved in an excess of carbonate of ammonium; in this solution no cloudiness should be produced by a drop of phosphoric acid.

It should be *cautiously* preserved.

Zincum chloratum.

[Chloride of Zinc]. Chlorzink.

Zincum muriaticum.

A white powder, which readily deliquesces in the air. It melts when heated, and is dissipated in white fumes, leaving a residue, which becomes yellow at a red heat. It is readily soluble in water, forming a somewhat turbid solution, which becomes clear on the addition of hydrochloric acid; this solution should not be rendered cloudy on the addition of alcohol. All the characteristic marks of the purity of chloride of zinc are similar to those of sulphate of zinc.

It should be *cautiously* preserved in well-closed vessels.

Zincum ferrocyanatum.

[Ferrocyanide of Zinc]. Ferrocyanzink.

Take of Ferrocyanide of Potassium *six parts*. . . . 6
Dissolve it in
Distilled Water *sixty parts*, ... 60
and gradually add a solution made of
Sulphate of Zinc *eight parts*, ... 8
Distilled Water *one hundred and eighty parts*. . 180

Let the mixture stand in a warm place that the precipitate may fall, and until the supernatant liquid has only an opalescent appearance. Then bring the supernatant liquid on a filter, and pour that which passes repeatedly back on the filter until the liquid runs off clear. Finally, transfer the precipitate to the same filter, wash it well with distilled water, and dry it at a gentle heat.

A white powder, insoluble in water, water of ammonia and diluted acids. When exposed to a red heat it leaves a residue of an alkaline reaction, which, when dissolved in hydrochloric acid, throws down a blue precipitate on the addition of ferrocyanide of potassium.

It should be *cautiously* preserved in a well-closed vessel.

Zincum lacticum.

[LACTATE OF ZINC]. Milchsaures Zinkoxyd.

In white, shining acicular crystals, or white crystalline crusts; or in the form of a very white powder. It is soluble in sixty parts of cold water, and in six parts of boiling water; insoluble in alcohol.

It must not blacken when concentrated sulphuric acid is poured upon it. Sixty parts of water should wholly dissolve one part of lactate of zinc upon the application of a gentle heat, forming a solution which reddens litmus paper, and has an acidulous, astringent taste, free from bitterness, and, on the addition of hydrosulphuric acid, yields a white precipitate; but it must not be rendered turbid by chloride of barium, nitrate of silver, or acetate of lead. The same solution gives, when mixed with carbonate of ammonium, a white precipitate, which should be soluble in an excess of the reagent. The solution thus formed should not become turbid on the addition of phosphate of sodium, but remain permanently clear.

It should be *cautiously* preserved in a well-closed vessel.

Zincum oxydatum purum.

[PURE OXIDE OF ZINC]. Reines Zinkoxyd.

A rather soft powder, becoming yellowish when heated.

Water that has been shaken with oxide of zinc, and filtered, is not rendered turbid by chloride of barium, or nitrate of silver, and should leave no residue when evaporated. It dissolves without effervescence in acetic acid, forming a solution which should not become turbid by water of ammonia in excess, but the solution yields, on the addition of hydrosulphuric acid, a white precipitate, which is soluble in hydrochloric acid.

It should be preserved in well-closed vessels.

Zincum oxydatum venale.

[COMMERCIAL OXIDE OF ZINC]. Käufliches Zinkoxyd.

[*Flowers of Zinc*]. *Zinkweiss. Flores Zinci.*

A white powder, becoming yellowish when heated, and dissolving readily and completely in acetic acid.

Dissolved in any diluted acid, on the addition of solution of caustic potassa, it throws down a white precipitate, which is entirely soluble in an excess of the alkaline reagent. It is employed merely in preparing Ointment of Oxide of Zinc, and for other preparations of zinc.

It should be preserved in well-closed vessels.

Zincum sulfocarbolicum.

[SULPHO-CARBOLATE OF ZINC]. Carbolschwefelsaures Zinkoxyd.

Phenylschwefelsaures Zinkoxyd. Zincum sulfophenylicum.

In transparent, colorless, rhombic prisms, having but a feeble odor of carbolic acid, or being entirely without smell, dissolving readily and wholly in water and alcohol.

The aqueous solution yields a precipitate on the addition of hydrosulphate of ammonium, and, when mixed with an excess of the reagent, the filtered liquid, when evaporated, leaves a residue, which is entirely dissipated by a strong heat. Its aqueous solution turns violet on the addition of a few drops of solution of sesquichloride of iron. Sulpho-carbolate of Zinc contains about fifteen per cent. of oxide of zinc.

It should be *cautiously* preserved in well-closed vessels.

Zincum sulfuricum.

[SULPHATE OF ZINC]. Schwefelsaures Zinkoxyd.

[*Pure White Vitriol*]. *Reiner weisser Vitriol. Vitriolum album purum.*

In colorless and inodorous, generally prismatic, crystals, slowly efflorescing in the air. It is soluble in equal parts of water; scarcely soluble in alcohol.

Its aqueous solution, on the addition of water of ammonia, yields a precipitate, which is entirely soluble in an excess of the reagent, and should not be colored when treated with hydrosulphuric acid.

It should be *cautiously* preserved in well-closed vessels.

Zincum valerianicum.

[VALERIANATE OF ZINC]. Baldriansaures Zinkoxyd.

In small white crystals, of a pearly lustre, having a greasy feel, and the odor of valerianic acid. It dissolves in ninety parts of cold, and in a less proportion of hot water; also soluble in alcohol.

It should yield valerianic acid, when water, mixed with a few drops of hydrochloric acid, is poured upon it. It is entirely soluble in an excess of water of ammonia, and the resulting solution should not be affected by chloride of calcium, nor by phosphate of sodium.

One hundred parts of Valerianate of Zinc should contain nearly thirty parts of oxide of zinc.

It should be *cautiously* preserved in well-closed vessels.

REAGENTS.

Acidum aceticum dilutum: DILUTED ACETIC ACID.

Acidum hydrochloricum: PURE HYDROCHLORIC ACID.

Acidum nitricum: PURE NITRIC ACID.

Acidum oxalicum: OXALIC ACID, *dissolved in twenty parts of Distilled Water.*

Acidum sulfuricum: PURE SULPHURIC ACID.

Acidum sulfuricum dilutum: DILUTED SULPHURIC ACID.

Acidum tannicum: TANNIC ACID, *dissolved in nine parts of Distilled Water, with one part of Alcohol.*

Acidum tartaricum: TARTARIC ACID, *dissolved in five parts of Distilled Water, when used.*

Æther: ETHER.

Ammonium carbonicum: CARBONATE OF AMMONIUM, *dissolved in five parts of Distilled Water.*

Ammonium chloratum: CHLORIDE OF AMMONIUM, *dissolved in ten parts of Distilled Water.*

Ammonium oxalicum: OXALATE OF AMMONIUM, *dissolved in twenty parts of Distilled Water.*

Amylum: STARCH.

Aqua bromata: BROMINE WATER. *Bromine is dissolved in forty parts of Distilled Water.*

Aqua Calcariæ: LIME WATER.

Aqua chlorata: CHLORINE WATER.

Aqua hydrosulfurata: AQUEOUS SOLUTION OF HYDROSULPHURIC ACID.

Argentum nitricum: NITRATE OF SILVER, *dissolved in twenty parts of Distilled Water.*

Argentum sulfuricum: SULPHATE OF SILVER, *dissolved in one hundred parts of Distilled Water.*

Baryum chloratum: CHLORIDE OF BARIUM, *dissolved in ten parts of Distilled Water.*

Baryta nitrica: NITRATE OF BARIUM, *dissolved in twenty parts of Distilled Water.*

Benzolum: BENZOL.

Calcaria sulfurica: SULPHATE OF CALCIUM, *a saturated aqueous solution.*

Carboneum sulfuratum: BISULPHIDE OF CARBON.

Charta exploratoria cærula: BLUE TEST-PAPER.

Charta exploratoria lutea: YELLOW TEST-PAPER.

Charta exploratoria rubra: RED TEST-PAPER.

Chloroformium: CHLOROFORM.

Cuprum metallicum: METALLIC COPPER.

Cuprum sulfuricum: SULPHATE OF COPPER, *dissolved in ten parts of Distilled Water.*

Ferrum sulfuricum crystallisatum: CRYSTALLIZED PROTOSULPHATE OF IRON *precipitated with Alcohol.*

Ferrum sulfuratum: SULPHURET OF IRON.

Hydrargyrum bichloratum: BICHLORIDE OF MERCURY, *dissolved in twenty parts of Distilled Water.*

Kali aceticum: ACETATE OF POTASSIUM, *dissolved in five parts of Distilled Water.*

Kali bichromicum: BICHROMATE OF POTASSIUM, *dissolved in ten parts of Distilled Water.*

Kali hypermanganicum: PERMANGANATE OF POTASSIUM, *dissolved in ten thousand parts of Distilled Water.*

Kali sulfuricum: SULPHATE OF POTASSIUM, *dissolved in fifteen parts of Distilled Water.*

Kalium ferricyanatum: FERRIDCYANIDE OF POTASSIUM, *dissolved in ten parts of Distilled Water, when used.*

Kalium ferrocyanatum: FERROCYANIDE OF POTASSIUM, *dissolved in ten parts of Distilled Water.*

Kalium iodatum: IODIDE OF POTASSIUM, *dissolved in twenty parts of Distilled Water.*

Kalium sulfocyanatum: SULPHOCYANIDE OF POTASSIUM, *dissolved in twenty parts of Distilled Water.*

Liquor Ammonii caustici: WATER OF AMMONIA.

Liquor Ammonii sulfurati: SOLUTION OF HYDROSULPHATE OF AMMONIUM.

Liquor Ferri sesquichlorati: SOLUTION OF SESQUICHLORIDE OF IRON, *diluted with five parts of Distilled Water.*

Liquor Natri caustici: SOLUTION OF CAUSTIC SODA, *diluted with two parts of Distilled Water.*

Magnesia sulfurica: SULPHATE OF MAGNESIUM, *dissolved in ten parts of Distilled Water.*

Natrum carbonicum: CARBONATE OF SODIUM, *dissolved in ten parts of Distilled Water.*

Natrum phosphoricum: PHOSPHATE OF SODIUM, *dissolved in ten parts of Distilled Water.*

Natrum subsulfurosum: HYPOSULPHITE OF SODIUM, *dissolved in ten parts of Distilled Water.*

Platinum bichloratum: BICHLORIDE OF PLATINUM, *dissolved in twenty parts of Distilled Water.*

Plumbum aceticum: ACETATE OF LEAD, *dissolved in ten parts of Distilled Water.*

Solutio Indici: SOLUTION OF INDIGO.

Spiritus: ALCOHOL.

Spiritus absolutus: ABSOLUTE ALCOHOL.

Stannum chloratum: PROTOCHLORIDE OF TIN, *dissolved in ten parts of Distilled Water, to which is added a small quantity of Hydrochloric Acid.*

Tinctura Iodi: TINCTURE OF IODINE.

Zincum metallicum purissimum: CHEMICALLY PURE METALLIC ZINC.

TABLE A.

Designating the largest doses (maximum doses), for an adult, which the Physician must not exceed in his prescription, when intended for internal use, except he adds the exclamation point (!).

Latin and English Names of the Medicines.	Grammes. For a single dose.	Grammes. Aggregate for a day.
Acidum arsenicosum: Arsenious Acid, . . .	0.005	0.01
Acidum carbolicum cryst.: Crystallized Carbolic Acid, ...	0.05	0.15
Aconitinum: Aconitia, ...	0.004	0.03
Aqua Amygdalarum amararum: Bitter Almond Water, ...	2.0	7.0
Aqua Lauro-Cerasi: Cherry-Laurel Water, . .	2.0	7.0
Argentum nitricum: Nitrate of Silver, . . .	0.03	0.2
Atropinum: Atropia, ...	0.001	0.003
Atropinum sulfuricum: Sulphate of Atropia, .	0.001	0.003
Auro-Natrium chloratum: Chloride of Gold and Sodium, ...	0.06	0.2
Baryum chloratum: Chloride of Barium, . .	0.12	1.5
Cantharides: Cantharides, ...	0.05	0.15
Codeinum: Codeia, ...	0.05	0.1
Coniinum: Conia, ...	0.001	0.003
Cuprum sulfuricum: Sulphate of Copper, . .	0.1	0.4
Cuprum sulfuricum pro emetico refracta dosi: Sulphate of Copper, as an emetic, in divided doses, ...	1.0	—
Cuprum sulfuricum ammoniatum: Ammonio-Sulphate of Copper, ...	0.1	0.4
Extractum Aconiti: Extract of Aconite, . .	0.025	0.1
Extractum Belladonnæ: Extract of Belladonna,	0.1	0.4
Extractum Cannabis Indicæ: Extract of Indian Hemp, ...	0.1	0.3

Latin and English Names of the Medicines.	Grammes. For a single dose.	Aggregate for a day.
Extractum Colocynthidis: Extract of Colocynth,	0.06	0.4
Extractum Conii: Extract of Conium, . . .	0.18	0.6
Extractum Digitalis: Extract of Digitalis, . .	0.2	0.8
Extractum Fabæ Calabaricæ: Extract of Calabar Bean, ...	0.02	0.06
Extractum Hyoscyami: Extract of Hyoscyamus, ...	0.2	1.0
Extractum Lactucæ: Extract of Acrid Lettuce,	0.6	2.5
Extractum Opii: Extract of Opium, ...	0.1	0.4
Extractum Pulsatillæ: Extract of Pulsatilla, .	0.2	1.0
Extractum Sabinæ: Extract of Savine, . . .	0.2	1.0
Extractum Stramonii: Extract of Stramonium,	0.1	0.4
Extractum Strychni aquosum: Aqueous Extract of Nux Vomica, ...	0.2	0.6
Extractum Strychni spirituosum: Alcholic Extract of Nux Vomica, ...	0.05	0.15
Folia Belladonnæ: Belladonna Leaves, . . .	0.2	0.6
Folia Digitalis: Digitalis Leaves, ...	0.3	1.0
Folia Hyoscyami: Hyoscyamus Leaves, . .	0.3	1.0
Folia Stramonii: Stramonium Leaves, . . .	0.25	1.0
Folia Toxicodendri: Poison Oak, ...	0.4	1.2
Fructus Colocynthidis præparati: Prepared Colocynth, ...	0.3	1.0
Fructus Sabadillæ: Cevadilla Seeds, ...	0.25	1.0
Gutti: Gamboge, ...	0.3	1.0
Herba Conii: Conium Leaves, ...	0.3	2.0
Hydrargyrum bichloratum corrosivum: Corrosive Chloride of Mercury, ...	0.03	0.1
Hydrargyrum biiodatum rubrum: Red Iodide of Mercury, ...	0.03	0.1
Hydrargyrum iodatum flavum: Green Iodide of Mercury, ...	0.06	0.4
Hydrargyrum nitricum oxydulatum: Subnitrate of Mercury, ...	0.015	0.06
Hydrargyrum oxydatum rubrum: Red Oxide of Mercury, ...	0.03	0.1

Latin and English Names of the Medicines.	Grammes. For a single dose.	Aggregate for a day.
Kreosotum: Creasote,	0.05	0.2
Lactucarium: Lactucarium,	0.3	1.2
Liquor Hydrargyri nitrici oxydulati: Solution of Subnitrate of Mercury,	0.1	0.5
Liquor Kali arsenicosi: Solution of Arsenite of Potassium,	0.4	2.0
Morphinum: Morphia,	0.03	0.12
Morphinum aceticum: Acetate of Morphia,	0.03	0.12
Morphinum hydrochloricum: Muriate of Morphia,	0.03	0.12
Morphinum sulfuricum: Sulphate of Morphia,	0.03	0.12
Oleum Crotonis: Croton Oil,	0.06	0.3
Opium: Opium,	0.15	0.5
Phosphorus: Phosphorus,	0.015	0.06
Plumbum aceticum: Acetate of Lead,	0.06	0.4
Radix Belladonnæ: Belladonna Root,	0.1	0.4
Radix Hellebori viridis: European Green Hellebore,	0.3	1.2
Rhizoma Veratri: White Hellebore Root,	0.3	1.2
Santoninum: Santonin,	0.1	0.5
Semen Strychni: Nux Vomica,	0.1	0.3
Strychninum: Strychnia,	0.01	0.03
Strychninum nitricum: Nitrate of Strychnia,	0.01	0.03
Tartarus stibiatus: Tartar Emetic,	0.2	1.0
Tinctura Aconiti: Tincture of Aconite Root,	1.0	4.0
Tinctura Belladonnæ: Tincture of Belladonna,	1.0	4.0
Tinctura Cantharidum: Tincture of Cantharides,	0.5	1.5
Tinctura Colchici: Tincture of Colchicum,	2.0	6.0
Tinctura Colocynthidis: Tincture of Colocynth,	1.0	3.0
Tinctura Digitalis: Tincture of Digitalis,	2.0	6.0
Tinctura Digitalis ætherea: Ethereal Tincture of Digitalis,	1.0	3.0
Tinctura Iodi: Tincture of Iodine,	0.3	1.2
Tinctura Opii crocata: Tincture of Opium and Saffron,	1.5	5.0

Latin and English Names of the Medicines.	Grammes. For a single dose.	Grammes. Aggregate for a day.
Tinctura Opii simplex: Tincture of Opium, .	1.5	5.0
Tinctura Stramonii: Tincture of Stramonium,	1.0	3.0
Tinctura Strychni: Tincture of Nux Vomica, .	0.5	1.5
Tinctura Toxicodendri: Tincture of Poison Oak, ...	1.0	3.0
Tubera Aconiti: Aconite Root, ...	0.15	0.6
Veratrium: Veratria, ...	0.005	0.03
Vinum Colchici: Wine of Colchicum, ...	2.0	6.0
Zincum chloratum: Chloride of Zinc, ...	0.015	0.1
Zincum lacticum: Lactate of Zinc, ...	0.06	0.3
Zincum sulfuricum: Sulphate of Zinc, ...	0.06	0.3
Zincum sulfuricum, pro emetico refracta dosi: Sulphate of Zinc, as an emetic, in divided doses, ...	1.2	—
Zincum valerianicum: Valerianate of Zinc, . .	0.06	0.3

TABLE B.

Containing the names of medicines, which are usually called poisons, and which must be preserved **very cautiously** *in closed apartments.*

Acidum arsenicosum: Arsenious Acid.
Aconitinum: Aconitia.
Atropinum: Atropia.
Atropinum sulfuricum: Sulphate of Atropia.
Coniinum: Conia.
Hydrargyrum bichloratum corrosivum: Corrosive Chloride of Mercury.
Hydrargyrum biiodatum rubrum: Red Iodide of Mercury.
Hydrargyrum iodatum flavum: Green Iodide of Mercury.
Hydrargyrum nitricum oxydulatum: Subnitrate of Mercury.
Hydrargyrum oxydatum rubrum: Red Oxide of Mercury.
Hydrargyrum præcipitatum album: Ammoniated Mercury.
Liquor Hydrargyri nitrici oxydulati: Solution of Subnitrate of Mercury.
Liquor Kali arsenicosi: Solution of Arsenite of Potassium.
Phosphorus: Phosphorus.
Pulvis arsenicalis Cosmi: Arsenical Powder of Côme.
Strychninum: Strychnia.
Strychninum nitricum: Nitrate of Strychnia.
Veratrinum: Veratria.

Other medicines, kept in the Pharmacies, which are of nearly the same therapeutical activity, must be likewise kept in the same closed apartments, according to the legal regulations for the preservation of poisons.

TABLE C.

Names of Medicines which must be kept **cautiously** *and separate from the others.*

Acetum Colchici: Vinegar of Colchicum.
Acetum Digitalis: Vinegar of Digitalis.
Acidum carbolicum crystallisatum: Crystallized Carbolic Acid.
Acidum chromicum: Chromic Acid.
Acidum hydrochloricum: Pure Hydrochloric Acid.
Acidum hydrochloricum crudum: Crude Hydrochloric Acid.
Acidum nitricum: Pure Nitric Acid.
Acidum nitricum crudum: Aqua Fortis.
Acidum nitricum fumans: Fuming Nitric Acid.
Acidum sulfuricum: Pure Sulphuric Acid.
Acidum sulfuricum crudum: Crude or Commercial Sulphuric Acid.
Acidum sulfuricum fumans: Fuming Sulphuric Acid.
Ærugo: Verdigris (Subacetate of Copper).
Aqua Amygdalarum amararum: Bitter Almond Water.
Aqua Lauro-Cerasi: Cherry-Laurel Water.
Argentum nitricum crystallisatum: Crystallized Nitrate of Silver.
Argentum nitricum fusum: Fused Nitrate of Silver.
Argentum nitricum fusum cum Kali nitrico: Nitrated Lunar Caustic.
Auro-Natrium chloratum: Chloride of Gold and Sodium.
Bromum: Bromine.
Cadmium sulfuricum: Sulphate of Cadmium.
Cantharides: Cantharides.
Cerussa: White Lead (Carbonate of Lead).
Chloroformium: Chloroform.
Codeinum: Codeia.
Cuprum aceticum: Acetate of Copper.
Cuprum aluminatum.
Cuprum oxydatum: Black Oxide of Copper.
Cuprum sulfuricum ammoniatum: Ammonio-sulphate of Copper.

Cuprum sulfuricum crudum: Crude or Commercial Sulphate of Copper.

Cuprum sulfuricum purum: Pure Sulphate of Copper.

Euphorbium: Euphorbium.

Extractum Aconiti: Extract of Aconite.

Extractum Belladonnæ: Extract of Belladonna.

Extractum Cannabis Indicæ: Extract of Indian Hemp.

Extractum Colocynthidis: Extract of Colocynth.

Extractum Colocynthidis compositum: Compound Extract of Colocynth.

Extractum Conii: Extract of Conium.

Extractum Digitalis: Extract of Digitalis.

Extractum Fabæ Calabaricæ: Extract of Calabar Bean.

Extractum Gratiolæ: Extract of Hedge-Hyssop.

Extractum Hyoscyami: Extract of Hyoscyamus.

Extractum Lactucæ: Extract of Acrid Lettuce.

Extractum Mezerei: Extract of Mezereon.

Extractum Opii: Extract of Opium.

Extractum Pulsatillæ: Extract of Pulsatilla.

Extractum Sabinæ: Extract of Savine.

Extractum Stramonii: Extract of Stramonium.

Extractum Strychni aquosum: Aqueous Extract of Nux Vomica.

Extractum Strychni spirituosum: Alcoholic Extract of Nux Vomica.

Faba Calabarica: Calabar Bean.

Ferrum iodatum saccharatum: Saccharated Iodide of Iron.

Folia Belladonnæ: Belladonna Leaves.

Folia Digitalis: Digitalis Leaves.

Folia Hyoscyami: Hyoscyamus Leaves.

Folia Stramonii: Stramonium Leaves.

Folia Toxicodendri: Poison-Oak Leaves.

Fructus Colocynthidis: Colocynth.

Fructus Colocynthidis præparati: Prepared Colocynth.

Fructus Sabadillæ: Cevadilla Seeds.

Gutti: Gamboge.

Herba Conii: Conium Leaves.

Herba Gratiolæ: Hedge-Hyssop.

Hydrargyrum chloratum mite: Mild Chloride of Mercury.
Iodoformium: Iodoform.
Iodum: Iodine.
Kali causticum fusum: Caustic Potassa.
Kreosotum: Creasote.
Lactucarium: Lactucarium.
Liquor Kali caustici: Solution of Caustic Potassa.
Liquor Natri caustici: Solution of Caustic Soda.
Liquor Plumbi subacetici: Solution of Subacetate of Lead.
Liquor Stibii chlorati: Solution of Chloride of Antimony.
Lithargyrum: Litharge.
Morphinum: Morphia.
Morphinum aceticum: Acetate of Morphia.
Morphinum hydrochloricum: Muriate of Morphia.
Morphinum sulfuricum: Sulphate of Morphia.
Natrum santonicum: Santonate of Sodium.
Oleum Crotonis: Croton Oil.
Oleum Sabinæ: Oil of Savine.
Oleum Sinapis: Volatile Oil of Mustard.
Opium: Opium.
Plumbum aceticum: Acetate of Lead.
Plumbum iodatum: Iodide of Lead.
Pulvis Ipecacuanhæ opiatus: Dover's Powder.
Radix Belladonnæ: Belladonna Root.
Radix Hellebori viridis: European Green Hellebore
Radix Ipecacuanhæ: Ipecacuanha.
Resina Jalapæ: Resin of Jalap.
Resina Scammoniæ: Resin of Scammony.
Rhizoma Veratri: White Hellebore.
Santoninum: Santonin.
Semen Colchici: Colchicum Seeds.
Semen Hyoscyami: Hyoscyamus Seeds.
Semen Stramonii: Stramonium Seeds.
Semen Strychni: Nux Vomica.
Spiritus Sinapis: Spirit of Mustard.
Sulfur iodatum: Iodide of Sulphur.
Summitates Sabinæ: Savine.
Tartarus stibiatus: Tartar Emetic.

Tinctura Aconiti: Tincture of Aconite Root.
Tinctura Belladonnæ: Tincture of Belladonna.
Tinctura Cannabis Indicæ: Tincture of Indian Hemp.
Tinctura Cantharidum: Tincture of Cantharides.
Tinctura Capsici: Tincture of Capsicum.
Tinctura Colchici: Tincture of Colchicum.
Tinctura Colocynthidis: Tincture of Colocynth.
Tinctura Digitalis: Tincture of Digitalis.
Tinctura Digitalis ætherea: Ethereal Tincture of Digitalis.
Tinctura Euphorbii: Tincture of Euphorbium.
Tinctura Hellebori viridis: Tincture of European Green Hellebore.
Tinctura Iodi: Tincture of Iodine.
Tinctura Iodi decolorata: Colorless Tincture of Iodine.
Tinctura Ipecacuanhæ: Tincture of Ipecacuanha.
Tinctura Opii benzoïca, Camphorated Tincture of Opium.
Tinctura Opii crocata: Tincture of Opium and Saffron.
Tinctura Opii simplex: Tincture of Opium.
Tinctura Resinæ Jalapæ: Tincture of Resin of Jalap.
Tinctura Stramonii: Tincture of Stramonium.
Tinctura Strychni: Tincture of Nux Vomica.
Tinctura Strychni ætherea: Ethereal Tincture of Nux Vomica.
Tinctura Toxicodendri: Tincture of Poison-Oak.
Tubera Aconiti: Aconite Root.
Tubera Jalapæ: Jalap.
Vinum Colchici: Wine of Colchicum.
Vinum Ipecacuanhæ: Wine of Ipecacuanha.
Vinum stibiatum: Antimonial Wine.
Zincum aceticum: Acetate of Zinc.
Zincum chloratum: Chloride of Zinc.
Zincum lacticum: Lactate of Zinc.
Zincum sulfocarbolicum: Sulphocarbolate of Zinc.
Zincum sulfuricum: Sulphate of Zinc.
Zincum valerianicum: Valerianate of Zinc.

Other medicines, occurring in the Pharmacies, which are of nearly the same therapeutical activity, must likewise be kept apart from the others, and in the same place with the medicines named in Table C.

SPECIFIC GRAVITIES OF LIQUID MEDICINES, AT 15° C. (59° F.).

Acidum aceticum dilutum: Diluted Acetic Acid,	1.040
Acidum hydrochloricum purum: Pure Hydrochloric Acid, ...	1.124
Acidum nitricum purum: Pure Nitric Acid, .	1.185
Acidum phosphoricum: Phosphoric Acid, . .	1.120
Acidum sulfuricum: Pure Sulphuric Acid, .	1.840
Acidum sulfuricum dilutum: Diluted Sulphuric Acid, ...	1.113—1.117
Æther: Ether, ...	0.728
Æther aceticus: Acetic Ether, ...	0.900—0.904
Chloroformium: Chloroform, ...	1.492—1.496
Glycerinum: Glycerin, ...	1.230—1.250
Liquor Ammonii acetici: Solution of Acetate of Ammonium, ...	1.028—1.032
Liquor Ammonii caustici: Water of Ammonia,	0.960
Liquor Ammonii succinici: Solution of Succinate of Ammonium, ...	1.050—1.054
Liquor Ferri acetici: Solution of Acetate of Iron,	1.134—1.138
Liquor Ferri sesquichlorati: Solution of Sesquichloride of Iron, ...	1.480—1.484
Liquor Ferri sulfurici oxydati: Solution of Persulphate of Iron, ...	1.317—1.319
Liquor Kali acetici: Solution of Acetate of Potassium, ...	1.176—1.180
Liquor Plumbi subacetici: Solution of Subacetate of Lead, ...	1.235—1.240
Liquor Stibii chlorati: Solution of Chloride of Antimony, ...	1.340—1.360
Mixtura sulfurica acida: Sulphuric Acid Mixture, ...	0.998—1.002
Spiritus: Alcohol, ...	0.830—0.834

Spiritus æthereus: Spirit of Ether, ... 0.808—0.812
Spiritus Ætheris chlorati: Spirit of Chloric Ether, ... 0.838—0.842
Spiritus Ætheris nitrosi: Spirit of Nitrous Ether, 0.840—0.850
Spiritus dilutus: Diluted Alcohol, ... 0.892—0.893
Tinctura Opii simplex: Tincture of Opium, . 0.978—0.982

ALCOHOLMETRICAL TABLE.

Proportion of Absolute Alcohol by Volume, and also by Weight, in 100 *parts of Spirit of different Specific Gravities, at* 15° C. (59° F.)

Specific Gravity at 15° C.	100 Vols. contain Alcohol.	100 Vols. contain Water.	Alcohol by Weight in 100 parts.	Specific Gravity at 15° C.	100 Vols. contain Alcohol.	100 Vols. contain Water.	Alcohol by Weight in 100 parts.
1.0000	0	100	0	0.9751	21	80.81	17.12
0.9985	1	99.05	0.80	0.9741	22	79.92	17.96
0.9970	2	98.11	1.60	0.9731	23	79.09	18.79
0.9956	3	97.17	2.40	0.9721	24	78.13	19.63
0.9942	4	96.24	3.20	0.9711	25	77.23	20.47
0.9928	5	95.30	4.00	0.9700	26	76.33	21.31
0.9915	6	94.38	4.81	0.9690	27	75.43	22.16
0.9902	7	93.45	5.62	0.9679	28	74.53	23.00
0.9890	8	92.54	6.43	0.9668	29	73.62	23.85
0.9878	9	91.62	7.24	0.9657	30	72.72	24.70
0.9867	10	90.72	8.06	0.9645	31	71.80	25.56
0.9855	11	89.80	8.87	0.9633	32	70.89	26.41
0.9844	12	88.90	9.69	0.9620	33	69.96	27.27
0.9833	13	88.00	10.51	0.9607	34	69.04	28.14
0.9822	14	87.09	11.33	0.9595	35	68.12	29.01
0.9812	15	86.19	12.15	0.9582	36	67.20	29.88
0.9801	16	85.29	12.98	0.9568	37	66.26	30.75
0.9791	17	84.39	13.80	0.9553	38	65.32	31.63
0.9781	18	83.50	14.63	0.9538	39	64.37	32.52
0.9771	19	82.60	15.46	0.9522	40	63.42	33.40
0.9761	20	81.71	16.29	0.9506	41	62.46	34.30

ALCOHOLMETRICAL TABLE.—*Continued.*

Specific Gravity at 15° C.	100 Vols. contain Alcohol.	100 Vols. contain Water.	Alcohol by Weight in 100 parts.	Specific Gravity at 15° C.	100 Vols. contain Alcohol.	100 Vols. contain Water.	Alcohol by Weight in 100 parts.
0.9490	42	61.50	35.18	0.8855	72	31.30	64.64
0.9473	43	60.58	36.09	0.8830	73	30.26	65.72
0.9456	44	59.54	37.00	0.8804	74	29.20	66.82
0.9439	45	58.61	37.90	0.8778	75	28.15	67.93
0.9421	46	57.64	38.82	0.8752	76	27.09	69.04
0.9403	47	56.66	39.74	0.8725	77	26.03	70.16
0.9385	48	55.68	40.66	0.8698	78	24.96	71.30
0.9366	49	54.70	41.59	0.8671	79	23.90	72.43
0.9348	50	53.72	42.53	0.8644	80	22.83	73.59
0.9328	51	52.73	43.47	0.8616	81	21.76	74.75
0.9308	52	51.74	44.41	0.8588	82	20.68	75.91
0.9288	53	50.74	45.37	0.8559	83	19.61	77.09
0.9267	54	49.74	46.33	0.8530	84	18.52	78.29
0.9247	55	48.74	47.29	0.8500	85	17.42	79.51
0.9226	56	47.73	48.26	0.8470	86	16.32	80.72
0.9205	57	46.73	49.24	0.8440	87	15.23	81.96
0.9183	58	45.72	50.21	0.8409	88	14.12	83.22
0.9161	59	44.70	51.20	0.8377	89	13.01	84.47
0.9139	60	43.68	52.20	0.8344	90	11.88	85.74
0.9117	61	42.67	53.19	0.8311	91	10.76	87.04
0.9095	62	41.65	54.20	0.8277	92	9.62	88.37
0.9072	63	40.63	55.21	0.8242	93	8.48	89.72
0.9049	64	39.60	56.23	0.8206	94	7.32	91.08
0.9026	65	38.58	57.25	0.8169	95	6.16	92.45
0.9002	66	37.54	58.29	0.8130	96	4.97	93.89
0.8978	67	36.51	59.33	0.8089	97	3.77	95.35
0.8954	68	35.47	60.38	0.8046	98	2.54	96.83
0.8930	69	34.44	61.43	0.8000	99	1.28	98.38
0.8905	70	33.39	62.50	0.7951	100	0.00	100.00
0.8880	71	32.35	63.58				

APPENDIX

BY THE TRANSLATOR.

THERMOMETERS.

The *Centigrade* thermometer, used in this work under the name of *Celsius'* thermometer, has been long used in Sweden, and is now most generally employed in scientific writings. It marks the freezing-point 0° (zero), and the boiling point 100°; the degrees being counted upwards and downwards from the freezing-point; the temperatures below 0° being indicated by the prefix of the negative algebraic sign (—), as in all thermometers.

In Fahrenheit's thermometer the freezing-point of water is placed at 32°, and the boiling-point at 212°; the number of intervening degrees being 180.

It is evident that 180 degrees of Fahrenheit are equal to 100 of the Centigrade scale, and that one degree of the first is equal to $\frac{5}{9}$ of a degree of the latter, or that a Centigrade degree is to a Fahrenheit degree as 1 is to $\frac{9}{5}$.

RULES FOR CONVERTING CENTIGRADE TO FAHRENHEIT DEGREES.

Double the number of Centigrade degrees, subtract one-tenth and add 32; or multiply by 9 and divide by 5, and add 32.

EXAMPLES.

$$15° \text{ C.} \times \tfrac{9}{5} + 32 = 59° \text{ F.}$$
$$-10° \text{ C.} \times \tfrac{9}{5} + 32 = 14° \text{ F.}$$
$$-20° \text{ C.} \times \tfrac{9}{5} + 32 = -4° \text{ F.}$$

In the formulas with the sign (—), the number must be treated as an algebraic negative quantity, and when multiplied by 9 and divided by 5, the *difference* between the quotient and 32 will either be the number of degrees above or below zero of Fahrenheit—above if less, and below if greater than thirty-two. See table on page 336.

FRENCH SYSTEM OF WEIGHTS AND MEASURES.

The French system of weights and measures is connected together in a manner far more philosophical than any other system; and, as it is the one generally adopted by scientific men on the continent of Europe, and is gradually being introduced into the writings of men of science everywhere, it is essential that the principles upon which it is based should be understood.

The introduction of the Metric System into this country had been long recommended, and in 1866 its use was authorized by Congress. To furnish a convenient standard of comparison, and render the public familiar with the new measures, it was also authorized that the new five-cent piece should weigh five grammes, and be one-fiftieth of a metre in diameter.

The standard of reference of the French Metric System is a measurement of one of the great circles encompassing the earth itself. The ten millionth part of a quadrant of the meridian constitutes the *unit* of the system. This quadrantal arc was fixed at 6213 miles and 1450 yards English measure; consequently the ten millionth part of this, called the METRE, is equivalent to 39.37079 English inches, nearly 3½ inches more than our standard yard, or a fraction of an inch longer than the second's pendulum. The cube of the tenth part of the metre was taken as the unit of the measure of capacity, and denominated LITRE. The weight of distilled water, at its greatest density (4° C. or 39.2° F), which this cube is capable of containing, was called KILOGRAMME, of which the thousandth part was adopted as the unit of weight, under the name of GRAMME. The multiples of these measures, proceeding in the decimal progression, are distinguished by employing the prefixes, *deca* (ten), *hecto* (hundred), *kilo* (thousand), and *myria* (ten thousand) taken from the Greek numerals; and the subdivisions, following the same order, by *deci, centi,* and *milli*, from the Latin numerals.

English writers have not agreed upon a uniform system of notation or abbreviation. The French write 35 metres 429 millimetres thus: $35^{\text{m}}\cdot429$, and 13 grammes 26 centigrammes, $13^{\text{gm}}\cdot26$. Some American writers have proposed to place the initial of the unit at the left of the numerical expression, as in our Federal money, thus: M35.429, and G13.26.

A period divides the unit and multiples from the subdivision, as seen in the figures of the following

TABLE OF WEIGHTS.

		Grammes.
1 Milligramme	= the thousandth part of 1 grm. or	0.001
1 Centigramme	= the hundredth " " "	0.01
1 Decigramme	= the tenth " " "	0.1
1 Gramme	= weight of a cubic centimetre of water at 4° C. (unit of weight),	1.0
1 Decagramme	= ten grammes, ...	10.0
1 Hectogramme	= one hundred grammes, . . .	100.0
1 Kilogramme	= one thousand grammes, . .	1,000.0
1 Myriagramme	= ten thousand grammes, . . .	10,000.0

RELATION OF THE METRICAL WEIGHTS TO TROY WEIGHTS, USED IN THE UNITED STATES PHARMACOPŒIA.

		Troy Grains.		℔	℥	ʒ	gr.
Milligramme	=	.0154					
Centigramme	=	.1543					
Decigramme	=	1.5434					
Gramme	=	15.4340					
Decagramme	=	154.3402	=	0	0	2	34.3
Hectogramme	=	1,543.4023	=	0	3	1	43.4
Kilogramme	=	15,434.0234	=	2	8	1	14
Myriagramme	=	154,340.2344	=	26	9	4	20

Metrical Weights.	Exact equivalents in grains.	Approximate equivalents in grains.
Milligrammes.		
1 =	.0154	$\frac{1}{65}$
2 =	.0308	$\frac{1}{32}$
3 =	.0463	$\frac{1}{22}$
4 =	.0617	$\frac{1}{16}$
5 =	.0771	$\frac{1}{13}$
6 =	.0926	$\frac{1}{11}$
7 =	.1080	$\frac{1}{9}$
8 =	.1234	$\frac{1}{8}$
9 =	.1389	$\frac{1}{7}$
Centigrammes.		
1 =	.1543	$\frac{1}{6}$
2 =	.3086	$\frac{1}{3}$
3 =	.4630	$\frac{6}{13}$
4 =	.6173	$\frac{7}{11}$
5 =	.7717	$\frac{3}{4}$
6 =	.9260	$\frac{9}{10}$
7 =	1.0803	1
8 =	1.2347	$1\frac{1}{4}$
9 =	1.3890	$1\frac{1}{3}$

Metrical Weights.	Exact equivalents in grains.	Approximate equivalents in grains.
Decigrammes.		
1 =	1.543	1½
2 =	3.086	3
3 =	4.630	4½
4 =	6.173	6
5 =	7.717	7½
6 =	9.260	9
7 =	10.803	11
8 =	12.347	12½
9 =	13.890	14

Metrical Weights.	Exact equivalents in grains.	Approximate equivalents in Troy Weights.
Grammes.		
1 =	15.434	gr. xv.
2 =	30.868	ʒss.
3 =	46.302	℈ij.
4 =	61.736	ʒi.
5 =	77.170	℈iv.
6 =	92.604	ʒiss.
7 =	108.038	℈vss.
8 =	123.472	ʒij.
9 =	138.906	℈vij.

Decagrammes.			Exact equivalents in Troy Weights. drs.	grs.
1 =	154.340	ʒiiss.	2	34.34
2 =	308.680	ʒv.	5	8.68
3 =	463.020	ʒviiss	7	43.02
4 =	617.360	ʒx.	10	17.36
5 =	771.701	ʒxiij.	12	51.701
6 =	926.041	ʒxv.	15	26.041
7 =	1,080.381	ʒxviij.	18	0.381
8 =	1,234.721	ʒxx.	20	34.721
9 =	1,389.062	ʒxxiij.	23	9.062

Hectogrammes.			Ounces.
1 =	1,543.402	℥iii ℈v.	3.2154
2 =	3,086.804	℥vj ʒiij	6.4308
3 =	4,630.206	℥ix ʒv.	9.6462
4 =	6,173.609	℔i ʒvij.	12.8616
5 =	7,717.011	℔i ℥iv.	16.0770
6 =	9,260.413	℔i ℥vij.	19.2924
7 =	10,803.816	℔i ℥x ʒiv.	22.5078
8 =	12,347.218	℔ij ℥i ʒv.	25.7232
9 =	13,890.620	℔ij ℥v.	28.9386

Metrical Weights.	Exact equivalents in grains.	Approximate equivalents in Troy Weights.	Exact equivalents in Troy Weights.
Kilogramme.			Ounces.
1 = . .	15,434.023 . .	℔ij ℥viij. . . .	32.1542
Myriagramme.			
1 = . .	154,340.23 . .	℔ xxvi. ℥ix ʒiv.	. . 321.542

RELATION OF TROY WEIGHTS (OF THE U. S. PHARMACOPŒIA) TO METRICAL WEIGHTS.

FRACTIONS OF A GRAIN IN MILLIGRAMMES.

Grain.		Milligrammes.	Grain.		Milligrammes.	Grain.		Milligrammes.
1/64	=	1.012	1/25	=	2.591	1/8	=	8.098
1/60	=	1.079	1/24	=	2.699	1/6	=	10.798
1/50	=	1.295	1/20	=	3.239	1/5	=	12.958
1/48	=	1.349	1/16	=	4.049	1/4	=	16.197
1/40	=	1.619	1/15	=	4.319	1/3	=	21.597
1/36	=	1.799	1/12	=	5.399	1/2	=	32.395
1/30	=	2.159	1/10	=	6.479			

GRAINS IN EQUIVALENT METRICAL WEIGHTS.

Grains.		Centigrammes.	Grains.		Decigrammes.	Grains.		Grammes.
1	=	6.479	6	=	3.887	16	=	1.036
			7	=	4.535	20	=	1.295
		Decigrammes.	8	=	5.183	24	=	1.555
2	=	1.295	9	=	5.831	25	=	1.619
3	=	1.943	10	=	6.479	30	=	1.943
4	=	2.591	12	=	7.775	40	=	2.591
5	=	3.239	15	=	9.718	50	=	3.239
						60	=	3.887

DRACHMS, OUNCES, AND POUNDS IN EQUIVALENT METRICAL WEIGHTS.

Drachms.		Grammes.	Ounces.		Decagrammes.	Ounces.		Hectogrammes.
1	=	3.887	1	=	3.1103	8	=	2.4882
2	=	7.775	2	=	6.2206	9	=	2.7992
			3	=	9.3309	10	=	3.1103
		Decagrammes.				11	=	3.4213
3	=	1.166			Hectogrammes.	Pounds.		
4	=	1.555	4	=	1.2441	1	=	3.7324
5	=	1.943	5	=	1.5551	2	=	7.4648
6	=	2.332	6	=	1.8661			Kilogrammes.
7	=	2.721	7	=	2.1772	3	=	1.1197

RELATION OF THE METRICAL WEIGHTS TO AVOIRDUPOIS WEIGHTS, AS STATED AND USED IN THE BRITISH PHARMACOPŒIA.

1 Milligramme,	=	0.015432 grs.
1 Centigramme,	=	0.15432 "
1 Decigramme,	=	1.5432 "
1 Gramme,	=	15.432 "
1 Kilogramme,	= 2 lb. 3 oz. 119.8 grs., or	15,432.348 "

The British pound contains 7000 Troy grains, and it is divided into 16 ounces, each containing 437.5 grains.

1 pound = 453.5925 grammes. 1 ounce = 28.3495 grms. 1 grain = 0.0648 grms.

MEASURES OF LENGTH.

		Metres.
1 Millimetre	= the thousandth part of one metre, or	0.001
1 Centimetre	= the hundredth " " " "	0.01
1 Decimetre	= the tenth " " " "	0.1
1 Metre	= the ten millionth part of a quarter of the meridian of the earth (unit of length).	
1 Decametre	= ten (10) metres.	
1 Hectometre	= one hundred (100) metres.	
1 Kilometre	= one thousand (1000) metres.	
1 Myriametre	= ten thousand (10,000) metres.	

Relation of the Metrical Measures to English Measures of Length, the Metre being at 32° and the Foot at 62°.

	English Inches.		Miles.	Fur.	Yards.	Feet.	Inches.
1 Millimetre =	.03937						
1 Centimetre =	.39371						
1 Decimetre =	3.93710						
1 Metre =	39.37100	=	0	0	1	0	3.371
1 Decametre =	393.71000	=	0	0	10	2	9.710
1 Hectometre =	3,937.10000	=	0	0	109	1	1.100
1 Kilometre =	39,371.00000	=	0	4	213	1	11.000
1 Myriametre =	393,710.00000	=	6	1	156	1	2.000

Table for the Conversion of Metrical into English Measures of Length.

Metrical to English.		English to Metrical.	
Millimetres to Inches.	Metres to Feet.	Inches to Millimetres.	Feet to Metres.
1 = 0.03937	1 = 3.2809	1 = 25.4	1 = 0.3048
2 = 0.07874	2 = 6.5618	2 = 50.8	2 = 0.6096
3 = 0.11811	3 = 9.8427	3 = 76.2	3 = 0.9144
4 = 0.15748	4 = 13.1236	4 = 101.6	4 = 1.2192
5 = 0.19685	5 = 16.4045	5 = 127.0	5 = 1.5240
6 = 0.23622	6 = 19.6854	6 = 152.4	6 = 1.8288
7 = 0.27559	7 = 22.9663	7 = 177.8	7 = 2.1336
8 = 0.31496	8 = 26.2472	8 = 203.2	8 = 2.4384
9 = 0.35433	9 = 29.5281	9 = 228.6	9 = 2.7432
25^{mm} = nearly 1 inch.		4 in. = rather more than 10^{cm}	

MEASURE OF CAPACITY.

1 Millilitre	=	1 cub. centim.,	or the	meas.	of 1	grm.	of water.
1 Centilitre	=	10 "	"	"	" 10	"	"
1 Decilitre	=	100 "	"	"	" 100	"	"
1 Litre	=	1000 "	"	"	" 1000	"	"

or one cubic decimetre and unit of capacity.

		English Cubic Inches.		Wine or Apoth. Measure.
1 Millilitre	=	.061028	=	16.2318 minims.
1 Centilitre	=	.610280	=	2.7053 fluidrachms.
1 Decilitre	=	6.102800	=	3.3816 fluidounces.
1 Litre	=	61.028000	=	2.1135 pints.
1 Decalitre	=	610.280000	=	2.6419 gallons.
1 Hectolitre	=	6,102.800000	=	26.4190 "
1 Kilolitre	=	61,028.000000	=	264.1900 "
1 Myrialitre	=	610,280.000000	=	2641.9000 "

The British Pharmacopœia estimates the Litre at 1 pint, 15 oz. 2 drs. 11 m. (imperial measure).

WEIGHTS AND MEASURES OF THE U. S. PHARMACOPŒIA.

One Pound, ℔	=	12 Ounces,	=	5,760 Grains.
One Ounce, ℥	=	8 Drachms,	=	480 "
One Drachm, ʒ	=	3 Scruples,	=	60 "
One Scruple, ℈	. . . .		=	20 "
One Grain, gr.	. . . .		=	1 "

One Gallon,	C	=	8 Pints,	=	61,440 Minims.
One Pint,	O	=	16 Fluidounces,	=	7,680 "
One Fluidounce,	f℥	=	8 Fluidrachms,	=	480 "
One Fluidrachm,	fʒ	. . . .		=	60 "
One Minim,	♏	. . . .		=	1 "

WEIGHTS AND MEASURES OF THE BRITISH PHARMACOPŒIA.

Weights.

1 Grain,	gr.			
1 Ounce,	oz.	. . . .	=	437.5 grains.
1 Pound,	℔.	= 16 ounces, . . .	=	7000 "

Measures of Capacity.

1 Minim,	min.		
1 Fluid drachm,	fl. drm.	=	60 minims.
1 Fluid ounce,	fl. oz.	=	8 fluid drachms.
1 Pint,	O.	=	20 fluid ounces.
1 Gallon,	C.	=	8 pints.

Measures of Length.

1 line	=	$\frac{1}{12}$ inch.
1 inch	=	$\frac{1}{39.1393}$ seconds pendulum.
12 inches	=	1 foot.
36 "	=	3 feet = 1 yard.

Length of pendulum vibrating seconds of mean time in the latitude of London, in vacuum at the level of the sea, . . . } 39.1393 inches.

Relations of Measures to Weights.

1 Minim is the measure of			0.91	grains of water.
1 Fluid drachm is the measure of			54.68	"
1 Fluid ounce	" " "	1 ounce or	437.5	"
1 Pint	" " "	1.25 pounds or	8750.0	"
1 Gallon	" " "	10 pounds or	70,000.0	"

°C.	°F.	°C.	°F.
0	32.0	60	140.0
10	50.0	61	141.8
15	59.0	62	143.6
16	60.8	63	145.4
17	62.6	64	147.2
20	68.0	70	158.0
25	77.0	80	176.0
30	86.0	85	185.0
33	91.4	95	203.0
35	95.0	100	212.0
40	104.0	110	230.0
42	107.6	115	239.0
44	111.2	118	244.4
45	113.0	120	248.0
46	114.8	170	338.0
48	118.4	180	356.0
50	122.0	200	392.0
56	132.8		
58	136.4		

INDEX

OF THE ENGLISH NAMES.

INDEX

OF THE LATIN NAMES AND SYNONYMS.

(The Synonyms are in Italics).

INDEX

OF THE GERMAN NAMES.

INDEX

OF SYSTEMATIC NAMES.

THE READER WILL PLEASE MAKE THE FOLLOWING CORRECTIONS:

Page 23.—14th line from top, for *discolors*, read *decolorizes.*

" 23.—21st " " " " *discolor*, read *decolorize.*

" 60.—2d " " " " *European Buckthorn*, read *Alder Buckthorn.*

" 171.—6th " " bottom, for *Sherry Wine*, read *Genuine White Wine.*

" 305.—9th " " " " *Aromatic Spices*, read *Aromatic Species.*

www.ingramcontent.com/pod-product-compliance
Lightning Source LLC
LaVergne TN
LVHW020118110826
845151LV00001B/199

* 9 7 8 1 4 2 5 5 4 2 4 0 5 *